The Art of
Hojo Undo

The Art of
Hojo Undo

POWER TRAINING FOR TRADITIONAL KARATE

MICHAEL CLARKE

YMAA Publication Center
Wolfeboro, N.H., USA

YMAA Publication Center
Main Office: PO Box 480
Wolfeboro, NH 03894
1-800-669-8892 • www.ymaa.com • info@ymaa.com

ISBN-13: 978-1-59439-136-1
ISBN-10: 1-59439-136-X

POD 1015

Publisher's Cataloging in Publication

Clarke, Michael, 1955-

    The art of hojo undo : power training for traditional karate / Michael
Clarke. -- Wolfeboro, N.H. : YMAA Publication Center, c2009.

      p. ; cm.

    ISBN: 978-1-59439-136-1
    Includes bibliographical references and index.

      1. Karate--Training. 2. Martial arts--Training. 3. Muscle strength.
I. Title.

GV1114.3 .C53 2009   2009933388
796.815/3--dc22   0909

Disclaimer: The author and publisher of this book will not be held responsible in any way for any injury of any nature whatsoever, which may occur to readers, or others, as a direct or indirect result of the information and instruction contained within this book. Anyone unfamiliar with the tools or exercises shown should exercise great care when commencing his own training routine. *Hojo undo* training is not suitable for children under the age of sixteen or adults who are unable to undergo regular martial arts training. If any doubts exist, consult a doctor before repeating the exercises found in this book.

Printed in USA.

Dedication

To Kathy, whose unselfish heart has shown me how to be a better man.

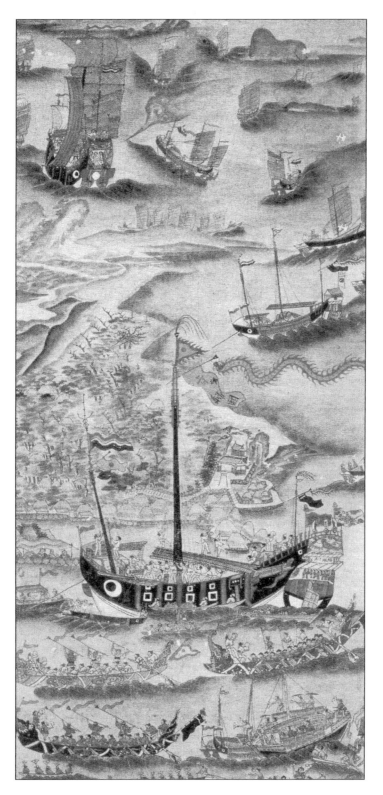

Okinawa's black ships traded across southeast Asia

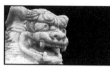

CONTENTS

Foreword by Tsuneo Kinjo, Kyoshi 8th Dan   ix

Foreword by Tetsuhiro Hokama, Kaicho 10th Dan   x

Foreword by Hiroshi Akamine, Kaicho 8th Dan   xi

Foreword by Patrick McCarthy, Hanshi 8th Dan   xii

Preface   xiv

Acknowledgments   xv

Photographic Credits   xvi

1 Introduction   1
Karate Beyond Okinawa   3

2 Preparation Exercises   9
About Junbi Undo   9
Junbi Undo Preparation Exercises   11

3 Lifting Tools   29
Makiagi – Wrist Roller   30
Chiishi – Strength Stones   34
Single-Handle Chiishi   40
Double-Handle Chiishi   48
Nigiri Gami – Gripping Jars   56
Tan – Barbell   65
Ishisashi – Stone Lock   77
Kongoken – Large Iron Ring   87
Tetsu Geta – Iron Sandal   98

4 Impact Tools   105
Makiwara – Striking Post   106
Tou – Bamboo Bundle   121
Jari Bako – Sand Box   126
Ude Kitae – Pounding Post   132
Kakite Bikei – Blocking Post   139

5 Body Conditioning Exercises 147

Ude Tanren – Two-Person Conditioning Exercises   147
Ippon Uke Barai – One-Step Blocking Practice   151
Sandan Uke Barai – Three-Step Blocking Practice   152
Wrist Rotation   154

6 Auxiliary Exercises 155

Push-Ups   156
Cat Stretch   157
Sit-Up and Punch   158
Drop and Thrust   159
Resistance Punching   160
Leg Resistance   161
Body Catch and Push   162
Heavy Squats   163
Leg Lift and Push   163
Stand-Ups   164
Fireman's Lift and Squat   165
Back Lift and Stretch   166

7 Other Tools and Methods 167

8 Comments on Hojo Undo from Okinawan Karate Masters 175

A Last Word   179
Endnotes   181
Glossary   189
Bibliography   193
Index   195
About the Author   201

Foreword
Tsuneo Kinjo, Kyoshi 8ᵗʰ Dan

There is probably no one in the world today who hasn't heard of *karate*. A number of fighting sports these days have incorporated *karate* techniques, but how many people can really say they know the difference between traditional *karate* and sports *karate*? *Karate* was the Okinawan people's sole weapon for self protection. In the words of *Goju ryu karate* founder Chojun Miyagi, "*Karate* is the ability to train your body to the point whereby you can overcome an opponent with one technique without the need for weapons." If you can't do that, you cannot protect yourself.

Sports *karate* has two branches, *kata*, which focuses solely on outward appearances and *kumite*, which is about winning and losing. Traditional *karate* however is completely different. The secret to traditional *karate* lies in daily training with the *makiwara, chiishi, nigiri gami, kongoken, ishisashi, kigu* training, and other *hojo undo*. All of this combines to train every part of your mind and body and helps foster a *bujutsu* spirit. Regular daily training is the true essence of traditional *karate*.

In this book, Mike Clarke has captured the secret of traditional *karate* power. As an Okinawan it makes me proud that Mike has taken the time to introduce to the world the essence of traditional *karate*. I hope that this book is well received by everyone throughout the *karate* world.

Tsuneo Kinjo, Kyoshi 8ᵗʰ *Dan*
Okinawa Goju Ryu Karate So Honbu, Jundokan
Asato, Okinawa

Foreword
Tetsuhiro Hokama, Kaicho 10th Dan

I want to offer my congratulations to Mr. Michael Clarke on the publication of his new book. Mr. Clarke loves Okinawa and has come to Okinawa many times for *karate* training and to learn more about *karate*'s history by continuing his own research. His detailed understanding of Okinawan culture is the reason this book can be written because it is about *hojo undo*, and this comes from our *karate* tradition.

To write a book like this about *karate* would be very difficult for an Okinawan *karate* teacher, but for a foreign *karate* teacher it must have been even more difficult and taken a great effort and a lot of patience. Mr. Clarke teaches *Goju Ryu karate* in Australia and has written other books about *karate*; he is respected by everybody. He is an honorable *karate* man of the next generation, teaching physical and mental techniques, and is my friend in *karate*. I highly recommend this book to everybody.

Tetsuhiro Hokama, Kaicho 10th *Dan*
International Goju-ryu Kenshi-Kai Karatedo-Kobudo Association
Nishihara, Okinawa

Foreword
Hiroshi Akamine, Kaicho 8th Dan

I first came to meet Michael through a series of interviews. He was doing research on *kobudo* weapons and wanted background for a number of articles he was writing for *Blitz Magazine* in Australia. We sat for several hours discussing the aspects of each weapon, what their origins were or could plausibly be, how they were used, what modifications were needed to make them truly effective fighting instruments, how they would be used in various situations, and any unique techniques which were associated with each. Throughout the interviews I was impressed with the effort he made to understand the answers.

When I saw the finished articles I was impressed with how he presented his research in context. He approached the topics as a person who had benefited from years of training; with his open mind, he was very quick to see how training in *kobudo* highlighted the underlying fundamentals of martial arts. While visiting, Michael noticed our array of *machiwara* and *chiishi*, and he asked how we used them in our training. That led to another pleasant conversation on training tools and techniques, which clearly demonstrated the depth of research he had put into this project even back then. I look forward to seeing what he has discovered in other *dojo* and how he writes about their training techniques and tools.

I recommend this text based on the quality of Michael's work with us on *kobudo*. I am sure it will be a valuable asset for learning how the tools are used as an extension of training the body and hardening resolve through strict application of effort and technique. These types of works are important in cataloging and transferring methods developed by our own teachers, and they make a fine addition to anyone's martial library.

Hiroshi Akamine, 8th *Dan*
President
Ryukyu Kobudo Hozon Shinko Kai
Tomigusuku, Okinawa

Foreword
Patrick McCarthy, Hanshi 8ᵗʰ Dan

The work which lies before you is not simply another "how to" book about *karate* but rather a penetrating look at Okinawa's principal fighting art, the culture in which it unfolded and one integral aspect of its practice, referred to as *hojo undo*. A rarely discussed aspect of our tradition, to the best of my knowledge Mike Clarke's work is the first book on this subject. A seasoned *karateka* and writer, the author's principal aim is to present this important practice in a historical context while revealing something of Okinawan *karate* culture, too. To this end I am confident that my colleague's publication successfully achieves his intended outcome.

Setting the contextual premise of *hojo undo*, the author has gone into great detail regarding the history of *karate* on Okinawa, but in a refreshingly bi-partisan manner. Like any true martial artist, Clarke is not interested in promoting the concept of *karate* "styles," but rather universal values, generic mechanics, and immutable principles instead. I'm certain that he has conclusively presented *hojo undo* as an integral if not natural part of training in the fighting arts—with or without weapons. He's also looked at how the idea of conditioning the body and mind collectively evolved alongside the fighting traditions from India through China and to Okinawa.

I particularly enjoyed the fresh way this author addresses the demise of "old-school" training through the introduction and rise of modern rule-bound practices—as one school of thought fell quietly dormant, another gathered momentum. Also, I am confident that Clarke's observations on how Japanese *budo* culture influenced this transformation and shifted its attention to *kihon, kata* (including incongruous application practices) and rule-bound *kumite* will explain an important yet rarely addressed aspect of how and why modern *karate* arrived in its present condition. Like any competent researcher, Clarke's reinforces his historical theory by referencing excellent English language sources dating back to the 1950s and 1960s. Drawing the reader's attention to both the past and present, I agree wholeheartedly when Clarke suggests that had *karate* been introduced to the West directly from Okinawa, rather than through the highly conformist Japanese culture, we would most certainly be embracing a creative art far more representative of Okinawa's old Ryukyu Kingdom Period and the holistic values it placed upon the living of daily life, rather than the rule-bound and overly ritualistic practices so widespread today.

Explaining the history and use of the most commonly found training equipment, the author discusses possible origins and shows how such apparatus can be easily constructed. This is particularly helpful for the reader interested in producing *hojo undo* equipment for the *dojo*. He's included many interesting stories and cited quotes from other writers' works that were appropriate. Including the lifting equipment, *makiage kigu*, two kinds of *chiishi, nigiri gami, tan, ishisashi, kongoken,* and *ishi geta*, Clarke's also written chapters on the impact equipment, such the *makiwara, tou, jari bako, ude kitae,* and *kakite bikei*. He's even included a chapter on *ude tanren* and a chapter on *junbi undo* (preparatory exercises) along with a dozen auxiliary exercises, which can be done when access to the tools is limited or nonexistent. Linking these exercises to techniques found in *kata*, and pointing directly to examples from both *Goju ryu* and *Shotokan*—two schools which perhaps best represent the principal traditions which form the mainstream of *karate* today—the author succeeds in offering far more than just an exploration into *hojo undo*.

With the absence of any work on *hojo undo*, *The Art of Hojo Undo: Power Training in Traditional Karate* is destined to become an instant success and I am pleased to be able to lend my name to its publication. Moreover, Mike Clarke's empirical experience and deep knowledge of both Okinawa's fighting arts and the culture in which it evolved makes him uniquely qualified to produce a book of this nature. Personally, I can't think of a single person anywhere in the world better suited to introduce this subject, and I highly recommend *The Art of Hojo Undo: Power Training in Traditional Karate* to teachers and students alike.

Patrick McCarthy, Hanshi 8th *Dan*
International Ryukyu Karate-jutsu Research Society
http://www.koryu-uchinadi.com
A link to the past is your bridge to the future

Preface

The photographs used throughout this book come from different times and from various sources and locations. They are in this book only to help inspire the reader who may be new to this aspect of *karate*. They do not always show the exercises being discussed. Construction advice is given for each tool and great care should be taken when making them. Build them as well as possible and keep safety at the forefront of any design and later use. Poorly made tools do little to improve your *karate* and places you in constant danger of injury. All weights and dimensions given in the construction advice are approximate, based on the tools used by me. As a result, each tool should be made to measure according to the person using it. If in doubt about either the construction or use of any of these tools, seek advice from a qualified teacher. The tools of *hojo undo* fall into two distinct groupings and have been presented this way: the first are "lifting" tools and the second are tools involving "impact."

Throughout the book I have written people's names in the Western way, for ease of reading and to avoid any misunderstandings that may arise for those unfamiliar with the Okinawan and Japanese custom of placing the family name first. I have also placed an English description next to Japanese words to ease the flow of information. I have deliberately used Japanese terminology throughout, as it was the language that introduced *karate* to the Western world and the language most non-Okinawans are familiar with today when discussing *karate*. Any mistakes in the information found in this book are mine and mine alone. Therefore I would ask only that they be viewed in the context of my humble effort to place before the martial arts public, information I believe is sorely needed.

Acknowledgments

This book could not have appeared before you without the help and support of a good many people, and it would be ill-mannered of me not to acknowledge their role in bringing this project to fruition. I am indebted in no small way to Ruarri Stewart, who gave so much of his time to interpret my primitive sketches and turn them into the first-rate construction and exercise drawings you see before you. It was a mammoth task, which he undertook with enthusiasm and diligence, and the results speak for themselves.

I am also grateful to those individuals whose research findings and their willingness to share them with others has allowed me to place *hojo undo* in its correct historical context. To Heiko Bittman, Charles C. Goodin, Tetsuhiro Hokama, Dr. Clive Layton, Patrick McCarthy, Mario McKenna, Graham Noble, and Joe Swift, I offer my sincere thanks.

To Hiroshi Akamine, Tetsuhiro Hokama, Tsuneo Kinjo, and Patrick McCarthy, all masters of their chosen martial art, for their generosity in writing forewords to this book and their support of my efforts, I can only express my deepest appreciation and thanks for taking time out of their busy lives to do this; their example as *budoka* serves as an inspiration to us all.

Also, I want to acknowledge the debt of gratitude I owe to the martial arts community of Okinawa. As a regular visitor to the island since 1984, I have never failed to be impressed by the warm and friendly character of the Okinawan people. Often on the receiving end of great kindness and hospitality outside the *dojo*, and meaningful insight inside of it—all bestowed upon me without hesitation or an expectation of something in return—I have yet to leave for home without feeling somewhat overwhelmed by the depth of their humanity. I hope in some small way this book shows a significant part of their cultural heritage and may be accepted as my attempt at *hachigo issu,** of giving something back for the magnificent gifts they have given to me in the form of *karate* and *kobudo. Nifee deebiru.†*

Because this is my fourth book I am sometimes asked, 'how difficult is it to write a book' and I have to say that the writing is not too difficult at all. However, writing a book that others want to read is a different matter. From idea to publication is a long and often tortuous process and few, if any, manuscripts flow onto a page and into a book unchanged. One person may write a book, but it is published through the efforts of many. I would like to take this opportunity to express my gratitude and offer my sincere thanks to all the people at YMAA publishing who worked on this project. I especially want to thank three key people, whose insight and talents have brought this book to publication.

First of all, David Ripianzi for his patience and skillful handling of my sometimes 'rustic' character traits. His encouragement to expand my original idea for this book gave

---

* *Hachigo issu* relates to the custom of giving something back in return for receiving a gift, or when an act of kindness has been shown towards you. It does not have to be (and is not meant to be), a gift or act of equal amount. The important thing here is the acknowledgment that you are mindful of the gift you have received, and so you show your appreciation.
† Thank you in the Okinawan dialect, *hogen.*

me the opportunity to learn a lot more then I thought I already knew, both about my self, and about how to write a book. I am truly grateful for his guidance.

I also want to thank Dolores L. Sparrow for taking on the 'challenge' of translating my manuscript from poorly written English into legible American, and for seeing something of value in the work that landed on her desk. Her work laid the foundations that the rest of the book was built upon. Dolores is an educator, whose influence has now spread to the other side of the planet.

Finally, this book as you see it today can be credited in no small way to the enthusiasm and efforts of its editor, Susan Bullowa. For a couple of months over the 2008 holiday season, she and I conversed and worked, and together we began to build the book you now hold in your hands. Her guidance (nurturing) gave me the confidence to abandon a few long held ideas, and to see possibilities that would have otherwise remained invisible to me. All this has led to a much better book than I had anticipated. "Thank you" doesn't quite cover it, but it is expressed with absolute sincerity.

Photographic Credits

Although the majority of images throughout the book are my own, some of the older photographs come from other people who have kindly allowed me to include them here. After considerable effort, I have been unable to trace or contact a small number of owners (the original photographers or others) of some of the images in the book. I apologize for this and request any unaccredited persons to contact me in writing. Upon proof of ownership, they will be properly credited (or their photograph removed if they wish) in any future edition. To the following, I am truly grateful: Kathy Clarke, Richard Barrett, Meitatsu Yagi, Tetsuhiro Hokama, Dennis Martin, Patrick McCarthy, Ron Ship, Anthony Mirakian, the Miyazato family, Kent Moyer, the Nagamine family, Graham Noble, Terry O'Neill, John Porta, the late Arthur Tansley, and *Karate-Do Magazine* in Japan.

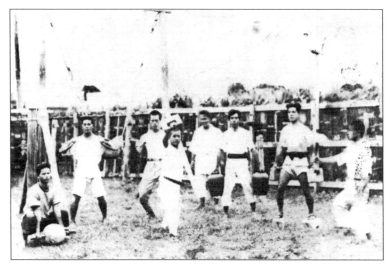

Hojo undo training at the Kenkyukai *dojo*, Okinawa c. 1928. Among those present in the photograph are Tokunori Senaha, Keiyo Madambashi, Chojun Miyagi, Jinen Shinzato, Seko Higa, and Seiko Kina.

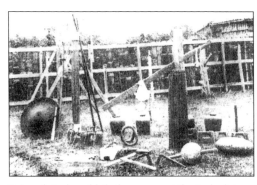

Hojo undo tools and *kobudo* weapons at the Kenkyukai *dojo*, Okinawa, c. 1928.

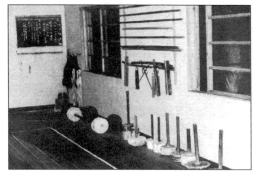

Hojo undo tools and weapons line the wall of Shinjo *sensei's dojo*. Photo taken c. 1973.

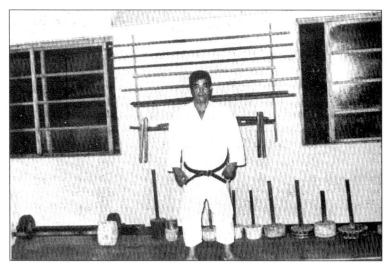

Masunobu Shinjo (1938-1993), a renowned teacher of *Goju ryu* and a firm advocate of *hojo undo* training. Photo taken c. 1973.

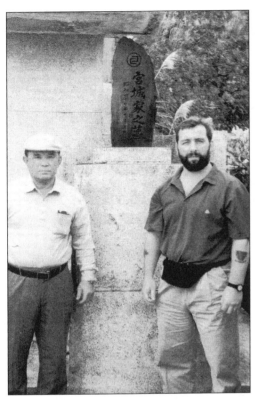

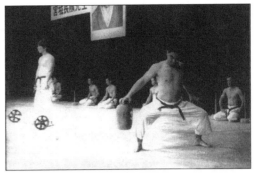

Jundokan students demonstrate *hojo undo* at the 20th anniversary demonstration commemorating Chojun Miyagi's death. Tokyo, October 1973.

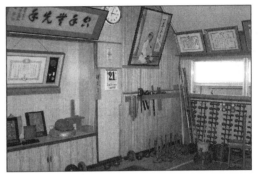

The author with his teacher Eiichi Miyazato (1922–1999) headmaster of the Jundokan *dojo*, at the grave of Chojun Miyagi (1888–1953) in central Okinawa, 1992.

Some of the *hojo undo* tools and *kobudo* weapons at Shoshin Nagamine's Kodokan *dojo* in Kume, Okinawa.

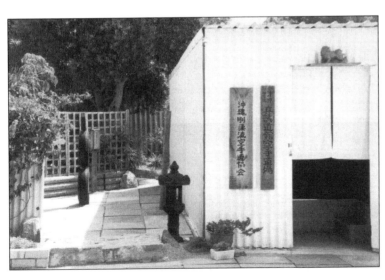

The original Shinseidokan *dojo* in Perth, Western Australia. Note the *hojo undo* tools in the small courtyard next to the *dojo*.

1 INTRODUCTION

On the island of Okinawa, since ancient times, people who practiced the fighting arts have lifted weights and struck inanimate objects to develop their strength and endurance. *Hojo undo*, or supplementary training, also called *kigu undo,* borrowed heavily from the martial traditions of China. In both cultures, it seemed only natural to condition, in tandem, the body and the mind in the pursuit of martial integrity. To this end people devised the many and varied tools we find today. Almost all of them were fashioned from common household items, everyday workplace objects, and things that came easily to hand. So many tools have been devised that it is beyond the scope of this book to include each and every one of them, although you will find within these pages all the most commonly used equipment and training methods. The Okinawans followed the example of their Chinese counterparts by using such tools and training drills to enhance their strength, and in doing so even introduced a few of their own. The *makiwara* as we know it today, for example, was developed in Okinawa and is now arguably the single best-known piece of *hojo undo* equipment in the *karate* world. Many years later, in the mid-1930s, the renowned *karate* teacher Chojun Miyagi integrated the *kongoken* into Okinawan *karate* after he visited the Hawaiian Islands in 1934.

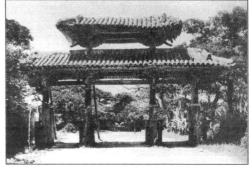

Old Shurei Mon (Gate of Courtesy). This gate, along with Shuri Palace, was destroyed during the battle for Okinawa, in April 1945. Today a modern replica stands in its place.

Regardless of which fighting methods the Okinawans practiced, with weapons or without, they always valued and utilized *hojo undo* in their training regime. Because of this, they became famous for not only their pugilistic abilities, but also for their astonishing strength and power in comparison to their size. In their quest to punch above their weight, martial artists in former times seemed to understand that the same trinity of body, mind, and spirit they needed to manipulate and control the various tools would also bring them the increased strength, confidence, and endurance they would need when facing an adversary.

The earliest mention of *karate* I have been able to uncover dates back to 1721 and comes from observations made by the Imperial Chinese envoy Hsu Pao Kuang in his *Record of Transmitted Facts of Chuzan* (Japanese: *Chuzan Denshinroku*), where he speaks of fists being used to punch (Bittman, 2005). A scant reference I'll grant you, but

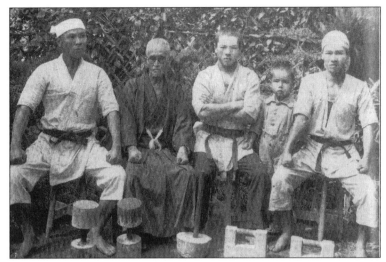

Chotoku Kyan and students c. 1941. Left to right: Jion Nakazato, Chotoku Kyan, Matsumoto, Nishihara, and Kurato.

clearly an indication of the fact that such activities were going on and in sufficient measure for him to take notice and include them in his notes. Forty-one years later, in 1762, Yoshihiro Tobe based his *Notes on the Great Island* (Japanese: *O'shima Hikki*) on the account given by envoys of the Ryukyu Kingdom who had been stranded in Tosa on their way to Satsuma. In it, the first written account of Okinawans training in a weaponless martial art is clearly pointed to when he notes: "A few years ago, Ko-shan-kin, who was skillful in the art of grappling, came from China with numerous disciples." The grap-

pling art of Ko-shan-kin he called *Kumiai Jutsu* and described it as a method of *Ch-uan-fa* (method of the fist). Over time, the memory of Ko-shan-kin's techniques have been preserved in the *Shorin ryu karate* tradition as the *kushanku kata*.

In his book, *(Concerning) Various Themes of the Southern Islands* (Japanese: *Nanto Zatsuwa*), written sometime between 1850 and 1855, Sagenta Nagoya offers his account and observations on the customs of the Ryukyu Islands. One tradition he draws the reader's attention to is the practice of

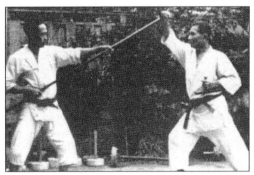

Eisuke Akamine (1925-1999) on the left, training *kobudo* with his *sensei*, Shinken Taira (1897-1970). Note the *hojo undo* tools in the background.

what he calls *Tsukunesu Jutsu*. We have only to look at the drawings accompanying his essay to see that *hojo undo* is an essential element in the martial art he is describing. For in his sketches we can clearly see a man training with a *makiwara*, and a second is conditioning the back of his fist (*uraken*) on a large stone tablet. The practice may go by a different name these days, but the image leaves little doubt that this was Okinawan *karate* he was writing about, and the drawings are clearly showing two types of *hojo undo*.

Karate Beyond Okinawa

The conditioning of the body cannot be done in isolation from the mind, because to condition one necessitates the involvement of the other. Discomfort and occasionally even real pain must be met, dealt with, and conquered. Taking it easy is not an option in the practice of *hojo undo*, because you are constantly pushing to stretch the boundaries of your limits and endurance. Within these pages, the reader will find information on how to construct each tool and training advice regarding their use, tools that are still used daily by followers of traditional Okinawan martial arts. However, this is not strictly speaking a training manual, and no scientific data or long explanations have been included. It is my view that science has intruded enough already in the study of traditional martial arts. No lengthy explanations have been given either, because experience with each tool will teach the lessons they have to offer, and in doing so, answer any and all questions you may have. Therefore, please treat this book simply as an introduction to an element of *karate* that is today largely ignored by the *karate* world outside of Okinawa.

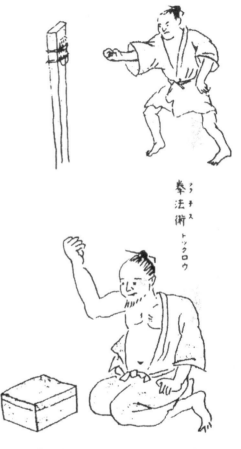

Drawings from the *Nango Zatsuwa* c. 1850 clearly showing *hojo undo* was an integral part of *karate* training.

It is interesting to note that the decline and subsequent disuse of *hojo undo* tools by the majority of Japanese and Western *karateka* seem to have paralleled the growth of sports *karate*. Just as the traditional methods of transmitting the art from one generation to the next were being discarded, a new idea of pitting one *karateka* against another in a sporting contest was on the rise. This shift in thinking gave increased impetus to the kind of *karate* training seen in most parts of the world today. Just as individual *karateka* were being encouraged to train hard to defeat others in the sporting arena, *karate* organizations began expanding in ever greater numbers to outdo their rivals. In Japan, training programs were set up specifically to provide professional instructors to other countries, and within a few short years of *karate* arriving in Japan from Okinawa, it was being disseminated to an unsuspecting world imbued with a distinctly foreign flavor, that of Japanese *bushido*. This shift in mentality changed forever the way *karate* was viewed in the West. In Japan, the term *bushi* meant *samurai*, but on Okinawa the term *bushi* is used to describe a gentleman skilled in both fighting and literature, someone who has become a living example of *bunbu ryodo*, the way of scholarship and the martial arts.

Traditional *karate* and *kobudo* training have always been about getting the better of our own negativity and returning our nature to a state of balance. It is the internal struggle with our sense of self while the learning of our martial art continues, that brings with it the dual rewards of intellectual enlightenment and the physical skills needed to defend ourselves. Modern *karate* tends to look elsewhere for a fight, away from the self and outward toward other people; *karate*, for many today, has become an external struggle (both physically and even economically) with those around them. How did this happen?

The earliest books on *karate* published in mainland Japan included *hojo undo* as part of the overall training. Kenwa Mabuni, an Okinawan and pioneer of *karate* in mainland Japan and the founder of the *Shito ryu* school of *karatedo*, wrote a number of volumes on the art of *karate*, including in them the same tools being discussed in this book. In his 1934 tome, *Karate Kempo Kobo Jizai*, and four years later, 1938, in *Kobo Kempo Karate-do Nyumon* that he co-authored with Genwa Nakasone, he looked at *hojo undo* training in some detail. Gichin Funakoshi, also Okinawan and the founder of *Shotokan karate*, felt, too, the need to include the use of *hojo undo* in his writings at that time and to this end included in his book, *Karate-do Kyohan*, detailed instructions on ways to construct a *makiwara*. Both men had been educated in the old-school ways of their island home. Nevertheless, among their Japanese students, their Okinawan training methods would all but vanish in less than two decades following their deaths.

Even before their passing, at the time *karate* was being established in Europe and America in the 1940s and 1950s, the tools of *hojo undo* had largely disappeared from the training most people were doing. Lip service was being paid to it, as can be seen by its inclusion in the written information available, but few people at that time, besides Okinawans, would have known of or understood its role in their overall *karate* education. In 1959 when E. J. Harrison, the well-known British writer and *judoka*, published *The Manual of Karate*, the fifth chapter addressed the subject of *hojo undo* or as he called it in the chapter heading, "Auxiliary Apparatus For Training." The book was actually no more than the amalgamation of two Japanese books already published, *Karate-do Nyumon* and another work by Reikichi Oya that Harrison simply mashed together and translated into English. He himself had no personal experience with *karate* training although he was an accomplished *judoka*. His many books on *judo* and *jujitsu* published in the first half of the twentieth century had made him the ideal person, in the eyes of his publisher, W. Foulsham of London, to author a book on this new martial art from Japan. I mention the book here only to inform the reader that even though few if any *karate* enthusiasts outside Okinawa were training with these tools at that time, books being published and about to be published over the following decade included *hojo undo* as a part of *karate* training and that, regardless of the reality on the ground, this trend in the available literature was set to continue for some time.

Fifteen years later in January 1974 when I began training in *karate* in Manchester, England, the use of these tools was gone altogether from the general *karate* training to which my contemporaries and I were being introduced. I became a student of Mr. David Vickers who taught *Tani Ha Shito ryu karatedo* under the auspices of the Shukokai Karate Union, an association that was, at that time, affiliated with the Shukokai World Karate Union organization founded in 1948 by Chojiro Tani (1921-1998) in Kobe, Japan. While attending Doshisha University in Kyoto, Tani had been a student of Chojun Miyagi for a short time and then went on to become a senior student of Kenwa Mabuni, the Okinawan responsible in large part for spearheading the introduction of *karate* in the Kansai (central) region of Japan. *Tani Ha Shito ryu* was considered revolutionary at the time of its conception. Chojiro Tani, a former schoolteacher, had taken his knowledge of *karate* and merged it with ideas based on the scientific analysis of body movement in sports such as golf and athletics. Concepts, such as kick-shot, shoulder-shock, and double hip twist, saw the punches and kicks of his *karate* take on a look and feel unlike those seen in other forms of *karate*. Mistakenly labeled as a style of *karate* designed specifically for sport, Tani's *Shukokai* organization did nevertheless begin to transform the competition scene wherever it made an appearance. The name *Shukokai* simply means an association of like-minded people training together. Although these days, many people use the name *Shukokai* to describe their *karate*, relatively few are following Tani *sensei*'s original teachings.

A few years after Harrison's book hit the shops, in 1962, Henri D. Plée[1] of France wrote an influential volume on the art titled, *Karate by Pictures*, published by W. Foulsham. Plée was Europe's leading local authority on *karate* at that time and was responsible for bringing to the continent the first Japanese instructors. In those days, France was the place to be for Europeans who wanted to study *karate* without making the epic journey to far-away Japan. The style of *karate* Plée taught was *Shotokan*, although by this time (early 1960s) it had already changed from the *karate* Gichin Funakoshi had introduced to the Japanese in 1922. Even though four whole pages of Plée's 1962 book (16-19) are given over to the *makiwara* and how best to train with it, no mention is made of the other tools. This section of the book is repeated again in his 1967 work, *Karate: Beginner to Black Belt*, also published by W. Foulsham. Interestingly though, in this later volume he included some extra information and some excellent photographs of the *makiwara* being used by one of Funakoshi *sensei*'s students, Mononobu Hironishi. Mention is also made, but only very briefly, of training with the *tetsu geta* (iron *geta*). This is done by way of two photographs and the captions that accompany them.

In 1966, one of Gichin Funakoshi's senior students in Japan, Masatoshi Nakayama, wrote the book, *Dynamic Karate*, published in Japan by Kodansha International Ltd. This work took on biblical status in the eyes of many Western *karateka* deprived of an oriental teacher and hungry for instruction from Japan. At the back of the book, the author again takes a glance at *hojo undo*. The *makiwara* receives the most prominent mention, with two versions of the tool discussed, plus how to make a pad as an alternative.

The use of a heavy kick bag is also well covered. Of more interest to me is the inclusion of a wooden club, similar to an oversized baseball bat, the iron *geta* (clogs), and an iron hand grip that looks exactly like an *ishisashi*. Rather disappointingly, no mention is made of how to use the iron hand grip shown in the photograph, and the heavy wooden club is depicted only in much the same way as *kendo* players would use the tool in their training, by continuously making the same overhead cutting action.

In his recently published memoirs, Masao Kawasoe,[2] now 8th *Dan* and a master of *Shotokan karate*, relates what life was like training in *karate* under the leadership of Nakayama *sensei* at that time. As a member of the famous, some would say "infamous" Takushoku University *karate* club, his *karate* training involved little *hojo undo* training in the Okinawan sense[3] apart from the *makiwara*, which he was expected to face on a daily basis. Although he did use the iron *geta*, he saw little of the other tools or training methods.

In 1967, Tatsuo Suzuki, a 7th *Dan sensei* of *Wado ryu karate* living in London, wrote his first book on *karate*, *Karate-do*, published in England by Pelham Books Ltd. A landmark for British *karate* students at the time, it too looked at *hojo undo* as part of traditional training, but as with the book by Plée published that same year, it made only a brief mention of the *makiwara* and the iron *geta*. Coincidence? Maybe, but I think all this points more to the fact that Japanese *karate* was now clearly heading in a different direction from that of its Okinawan predecessor.

Meanwhile, across the Atlantic, in Rutland, Vermont, a book had been published in 1963 that showed the Western enthusiast, I think for the first time, what *karate* training was like from the Okinawan perspective. The publication of *The Way of Karate* by George E. Mattson[4] was a seminal moment in Western *karate* literature. Quite simply, nothing like it in depth or scope had been written by a Western student of either Okinawan or Japanese *karate* at that time. Even the *kanji* (Chinese characters) embossed in gold on a hardback black cover were written in the old Okinawan way that read *Toudi*. This was a mark of respect toward China used throughout the Ryukyu Islands that would soon go the same way as many of the tools and training methods used on Okinawa, once the nationalistic fervor gripping Japan in the early decades of the twentieth century found its way into the *dojo of karate*.

First-generation Japanese *karate* teachers never really valued the role *hojo undo* played in their students' overall *karate* training. Like the individual investigation of the *kata* through *bunkai, oyo,* and *tagumi* drills, they simply neglected it. Over the next four decades, from the 1920s to the 1960s, *hojo undo* fell from use, with the *makiwara* being the only remnant of it to survive to any degree in Japanese *karate* today. On Okinawa, however, *hojo undo* has continued to play a leading role in the *karate* education of its young men and women. Whereas the Japanese turned *karate* into a study of the three K's (*kihon, kata,* and *kumite*), the Okinawans had always pursued *karate* through a different route. For them *karate* training begins with *junbi undo* (preparation exercises), followed by *hojo undo* (conditioning exercises), then *kata* (prearranged strategy training in thin air), and finally *bunkai* (the fighting application of the *kata's* strategy on a training partner). While the Japanese have based their *karate* on the three legs, of *kihon* (basic techniques), *kata* (solo tactical training) and *kumite* (prearranged and freestyle sparring), Okinawan *karate* has always stood upon four legs: preparation, strength, strategy, and application. This book deals primarily with the second of these—*hojo undo*, the building of physical and mental strength through conditioning. However, it will also examine *junbi undo*, exercises done to prepare the body for training.

Kanryo Higaonna (1853-1915)[5] left behind the following advice for those training with the tools of *hojo undo*:

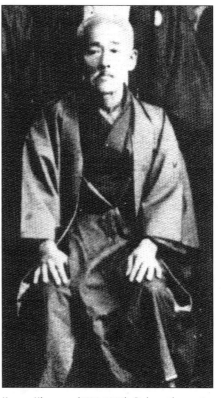

The results of your effort are cumulative:
- Never rush or show off.
- Train in accordance with your ability.
- Repeat each exercise until exhaustion, and build intensity gradually.

This advice has stood the test of time and is as relevant today as it was when he first gave it more than a century ago. The third piece of advice may need some clarification however. The exhaustion Higaonna *sensei* is referring to here does not mean that we need to reach a point where we fall over. Rather it means we must not stop simply because we begin to suffer a little from fatigue or discomfort.

Kanryo Higaonna (1853-1915). Perhaps the most famous exponent of *Naha-te* style *karate*, and the teacher of Chojun Miyagi, the founder of *Goju ryu*.

Ideally, training should be conducted under the guidance of a qualified teacher, remembering always that the key to benefiting from this form of activity is honesty and endurance. If a teacher cannot be found, the information that follows will help point the reader in the direction of self-discovery. Be patient, construct the tools with care and with an eye to safety, and be satisfied to gain your skills slowly. You should be aiming to build confidence through conditioning, and the gaining of such things cannot be rushed. The weight of each tool should be tailored to suit the user. Heavier is not always better. Too heavy and the exercises cannot be done; too light and little benefit is gained. If possible make your own tools, but if this is not possible, obtain weights that will test your endurance. Above all, be honest in your efforts and balanced in your expectations.

"Lift things properly; hit things with care."

The above maxim should be at the forefront of your mind when embarking upon the study of traditional Okinawan *hojo undo*. Find your limit with each tool and exercise, and then carefully and methodically push that limit further and further. In doing so, you will learn much about yourself and who you really are. Initially, it would appear our bodies are the focal point of the challenge we accept when we begin *hojo undo*. Once the serious training begins, it soon becomes clearly aimed at our own inner spirit. Make no mistake about it; these tools, if seriously worked with will bring you face to face with your real self. The question is will you like the person you meet?

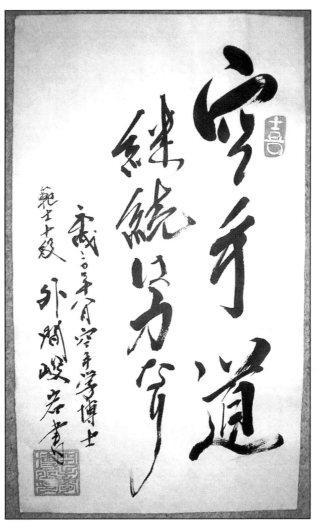

"Karatedo—continuation is powerful." Written by Tetsuhiro Hokama and given by him as a gift to the author. Author's private collection.

2 PREPARATION EXERCISES

About Junbi Undo

In an Okinawan *karate dojo*, warming-up exercises are known as *junbi undo,* preparation exercises. Within many Western schools of *karate* today, the warm-up exercises often have little in common with the mental activity that follows, neither do they always relate particularly well to the physical demands placed upon the specific muscle groups and tendons throughout the body that are about to be used in the *karate* training itself. While it is not my intention to deny the importance of warming up before *karate* training of any sort begins in earnest, it has to be said that the activities engaged in under this banner can often fall short when it comes to the question of preparing the body and mind for the demands of *karate*. While aerobic fitness and muscular strength are no doubt important, the strong body and calm mind required in traditional *karate* is based on the understanding of your body weight and how, through the connection with the ground and a calm and focused mind, that body weight can be best used to deal with and manipulate the force of an attack. While all hell may be going on around us, we strive to remain calm inside. In *karate,* we try to be the eye of the storm.

Within the *Goju ryu* tradition of Okinawan *karate*, a series of exercises have been handed down since the days of Chojun Miyagi, the tradition's founder. These exercises are intended to not only warm up the body, making it ready for training, but also to engage the particular muscles and tendons used in the various techniques of *karate*. They also play an additional role of focusing the mind on a particular part of the body as the routine is worked through, thus giving an early appreciation for some of the postures and "feelings" you are searching for in your *karate* technique. Because almost all of the techniques of *Goju ryu karate* are shared to some extent by other schools of martial arts, this set of *junbi undo* exercises should not be considered as being solely beneficial to *Goju ryu* practitioners alone.

In the main, there are two kinds of *junbi undo* exercises. The first stretches the muscles and tendons and loosens up the joints, which helps to promote suppleness and increase the range of motion in the moving parts of the body. This group begins to stir the blood and raise the body's temperature. The second group of exercises is done to build strength and stamina in the major muscle groups of the body and to increase your mental powers of endurance. Over time, these two forms of *junbi undo* combined enables the techniques of *karate* to be performed well within the range of the *karateka's* mental strength and physical suppleness. This in turn allows him to move freely and without the stresses imposed on a less supple or healthy body. The mind as well, familiar with the limits of the body, is calm and more able to achieve that relaxed state of concentration needed to deal successfully with conflict.

Beginning with the toes and working vertically up through the body to the neck, the first set of exercises is an excellent way to prepare both physically and mentally for the rigors of the training to come and to point your attention directly toward specific postures and positions encountered later in the actions of *karate*. These exercises, or something like them, should be considered as much a part of your *karate* training as a block, a punch, or a kick. What follows are the drills I teach and are practiced in my *dojo* before every training session. Even when the entire training is given over to *hojo undo*, these exercises are still done because students should never attempt to lift heavy weights from scratch without preparing their body and mind in some way first. To do so is to invite the possibility of torn muscles, tendons, or perhaps even something worse. The fibers of the muscles work better when prepared; so remember, you shock them into activity at your peril. All these exercises should be considered general warming up drills, albeit specific to *karate*. To improve your flexibility and muscular strength to their full potential, you should seek expert guidance from a qualified teacher of yoga, gymnastics, or weightlifting.

Junbi Undo Preparation Exercises

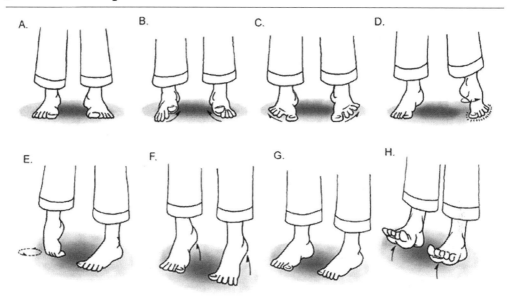

A. B. C. D.

E. F. G. H.

Junbi-Undo 1

Begin by standing in *heiko dachi* (natural stance, Figure A), resting the hands on the hips, and focusing your attention on the soles of the feet (*teisoku*). Spread the toes as widely as possible and try to make as much surface contact with the ground as you can.

From here lift up your big toe (Figure B) and hold for a second before returning it to the ground, gripping the floor, and lifting the smaller toes (Figure C) off the ground. This exchange is repeated at least ten times. The big toe up position is the same posture made with the foot when kicking *yoko geri* (side kick). With the big toe down and the small toes up, this foot position is used in *kata* when turning front on from a sideward stance, as in the *gekisai kata*, i.e., when moving from *heiko dachi* to *sanchin dachi* after the *jodan shuto uchi* (head height open-hand strike). It is also found toward the end of the *kata saifa* when moving on from the second *chudan ura zuki* into *sanchin dachi*, to throw *hidari jodan gyaku zuki* (left side head-height punch).

Standing in *heiko dachi* (Figure A) and placing your weight on one leg, raise the opposite heel and grip the floor with the toes with as much strength as possible. Twist the heel inward toward the standing leg (Figure D), but do not allow the toes to lose their grip; hold for four or five seconds before releasing the tension. This twisting exercise should be repeated at least ten times with each foot. Over time, this drill increases the strength of the toes and improves their overall dexterity. This is important in *karate*, as often within *kata* subtle control tactics using the toes are employed.

One example occurs immediately after the kicks in the *gekisai kata*, and in the *Goju ryu kata suparinpei* where they precede the *awase zuki* (double punch) is yet another. In these and other *kata*, the toes are placed on the opponent's foot to keep him from retreating and to hold him there for the strike that follows. During this time, the big toe is used to apply pressure on a vital spot just above the opponent's toes (*kori*).

Placing your body weight on one leg, roll the toes of the opposite foot back and forth on the floor before making a circular motion (Figure E). Allow some weight to be brought to bear on the toes being rolled and take care to roll the big toe. This exercise increases your awareness of the toes and improves the overall dexterity of the big toe, a weapon so often left out of the *karate* arsenal, and yet, one that can have a mind-numbing effect when applied correctly as described in the previous exercise. Our big toe also provides us with the ability to balance properly and our understanding of its relationship with the ground is vital for our stability.

With the hands resting on the hips, raise the body up onto the balls of the feet (*koshi*) and hold for two or three seconds (Figure F). This posture works the tendon at the back of the ankle (Achilles tendon), stretches the calf muscles, and aids in the acquisition of good balance.

Placing the feet back on the floor (Figure G), rock backward on the heels (Figure H) before returning to the original position on the balls of the feet. Warming up the tendons and calf muscles of the leg, the first posture on the balls of the feet is also the foot position found in a *karate* front kick (*mae geri*). When on the heels, this foot position is found in the *Goju ryu kata seisan*, toward the end when kicking with the heel into the lower torso or bladder of an opponent (*kakato geri*). In the *Shotokan kata unsu*, this kind of kick is also used to great effect about two-thirds of the way through the *kata*,[6] although in that particular school of *karate* the technique is also known as *kesage geri*.

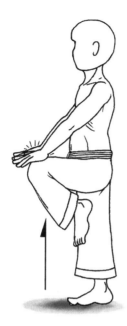
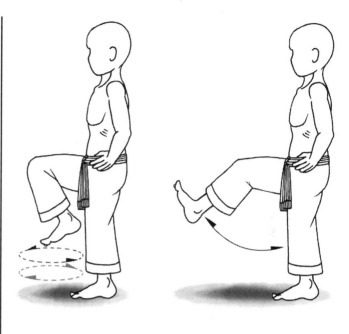

Junbi-Undo 2

Keeping the armpits closed tightly, hold the arms out in front of the body with the palms of the hands open and firm. Springing off the floor with the ankles, shoot the knees, alternately, into the open hands in a steady and rhythmical way making as much impact with the palm of the hand as possible. This movement not only prepares the legs for action later in the *karate* training proper, but also helps spotlight the actual mechanics involved in the execution of a kick with the knee (*heiza geri*).

Junbi-Undo 3

Returning the hands to the hips, stand on the left leg and raise the right knee so that the thigh is level; doing this helps develop balance. Rotate the ankle, first clockwise and then counterclockwise. Then flick the bottom part of the leg out as if kicking. Keep the leg relaxed while you do this and remember to form the foot properly as if doing a *karate* front kick (*mae geri*). Repeat this by standing on the right leg and raising the left knee.

A. 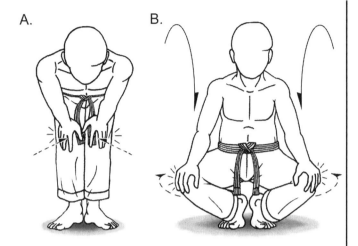 B.

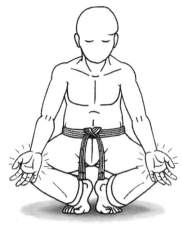

Junbi-Undo 4

Place the feet together with the heels touching and the toes apart making a V-shape with the feet (*musubi dachi*). Leaning forward, the hands are placed on the knees, where a little pressure is brought to bear to push them backward (Figure A). At this point, be sure the toes, especially the big toe, stay firmly on the ground, gripping the floor. The big toe provides us with the ability to balance properly, and a strong connection to the ground with this particular digit is therefore essential.

Bend the knees and drop the body down into a squatting position, keeping the back straight and the knees out to the sides as the heels leave the floor (Figure B). Remain in this posture for a few seconds before returning to the starting position. The bending and standing is repeated at least ten times, and care should be taken not to over-extend the knee joint by dropping too quickly into the squat. The hands remain on the knees throughout.

Junbi-Undo 5

On the final squat, hold for at least thirty seconds. Push the knees open and back, and keep the back straight: now close your eyes. After thirty seconds, open your eyes and stand up. This exercise helps develop balance while strengthening the toes and is exactly the posture (stance) required in the *Goju ryu kata kururunfa.* Toward the end of the *kata*, a 180-degree turn is performed bringing the *karateka* into *musubi dachi* (V-shaped stance) before dropping immediately into *koshi dachi* (squatting stance—standing on the balls of the feet). In the *kata,* this stance facilitates a throwing technique.

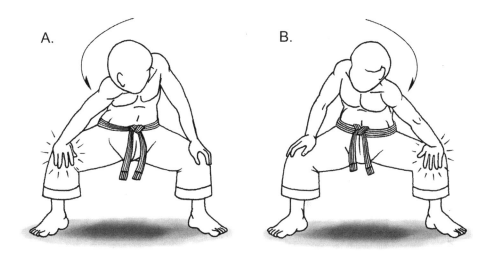

A.

B.

Junbi-Undo 6

Step out into *shiko dachi* (low stance) and place the hands on the inside of the thighs close to the knees. Drop the right shoulder forward, turn the head gently, and look to the left (Figure A). The right arm now pushes the right leg backward while the left arm checks the left leg from moving forward. Again, take care to keep the toes of both feet firmly gripping the floor throughout this exercise.

The stretch should be felt along the top of the inner thigh and should be held for several seconds before switching over and repeating on the opposite side of the body (Figure B).

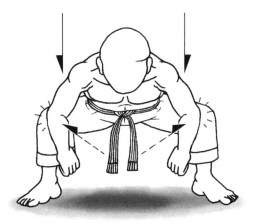

Junbi-Undo 7

Staying in *shiko dachi*, run both forearms down the inside of the legs until the elbows are slightly above the knees. Bring an equal pressure to bear on both legs to push them apart. With the toes gripping the floor, hold the chest up, as upright as possible, to maximize the stretch on the legs. Hold for at least ten seconds.

A timely reminder here—all stretches should be done with care and never rushed. Regardless of how flexible you might be, never drop into or come out of a stretch quickly. Always perform these actions slowly and methodically, and take care of your body.

When moving in *shiko dachi* (low stance), it is important not to lean with the shoulders first or to simply spin one leg around the other. Although there are some occasions where a spin is used, it is specific to the techniques being performed. Moving incorrectly in relation to the technique we are trying to do takes away control and the loss of control hinders our ability to affect the outcome properly, as well as the opportunity to adapt should the need arise. In this case, the body should remain upright while the weight transfer is taken care of by the legs when the "stepping" leg pushes the weight onto the "standing" leg before moving quickly to its next location. The result of moving from one posture to another, regardless of which method is being employed, should be predictable and never left to chance. Along with poor control of our own body comes a

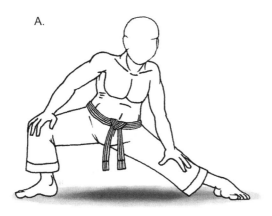

A.

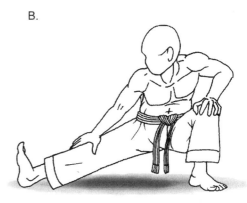

B.

Junbi-Undo 8

Lean onto the right leg and keep the left leg stretched out, with the foot and toes flat on the ground (Figure A). Rest the hands on the knees and try to maintain an image of the calf muscles being stretched by your posture. Without raising the body, move across onto the opposite leg, not by leaning, but by isolating the leg muscles and making the bent leg move the weight of the body across to the other side in as level a manner as possible. The idea is to recognize the exchange of your body weight from one leg to the other. This "feeling" is necessary in many *Goju ryu kata*, but particularly so in the *kata seiyunchin*. Hold the posture on either side for several seconds before moving back across in a steady manner. Ten repetitions on both sides gives the legs a good workout.

Moving directly on from the previous exercises and into this one, drop the body down into a lower (squatting) position and allow the foot of the outstretched leg to rest on the heel with the toes pointing upward, while keeping the foot of the squatting leg flat on the floor (Figure B). The stretch has moved now from the lower leg to the upper leg and with the lower center of gravity now involved, the feeling of transferring your weight increases; doing the exercise correctly strengthens the legs.

diminished ability to control someone else. It is important to remember that at the core of *karate* training is the challenge to control ourselves first. This speaks to our mind as well as our body and perhaps sheds light on why complete mastery of *karate* is an achievement accomplished by so few.

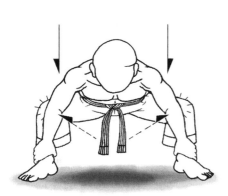

Junbi-Undo 9

With the legs having now had a good stretch, return to *shiko dachi* once more; place the elbows on the inside of the knees and push backward, remembering to keep the body as upright as possible and to grip the floor with the toes. Extra leverage may be gained by grasping the ankles with the hands.

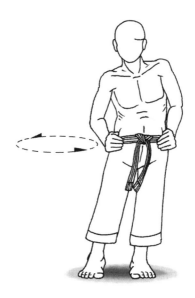

Junbi-Undo 10

Standing in *heiko dachi* (natural stance) with the hands resting lightly on the hips, rotate the hips in a circular action. Try to keep the ankles and shoulders in line and confine the movement to the central part of the body, minimizing as much as possible any movement of the shoulders; rotate the hips both clockwise and counterclockwise.

Within *Goju ryu karate* there is a method of turning that requires a strong twisting action, and this can be seen in the *kata*: *sanchin dai ni, saifa, seiyunchin, sanseiru, seipai, seisan* and *suparinpei*, where the successful execution of the technique immediately following the turn is directly linked to the amount of torque built up in the body immediately prior to the turn. If the shoulders and the hips twist on a different axis during the turn, then the transfer of energy is lost while the body becomes unstable and loss of balance occurs. Under these circumstances, the technique is almost certain to fail.

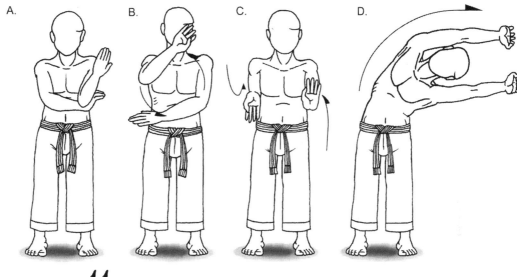

A. B. C. D.

Junbi-Undo 11

Standing in *heiko dachi* (natural stance) hold the left arm in a *chudan haito uke* (mid-level thumb-edge hand block) posture (Figure A) and support it by placing the right hand, palm facing down, under the elbow. From there inhale deeply through the nose while you perform *mawashi uke* (circular block, Figure B) and come to the position seen in Figure C.

Keeping the body and head facing forward, bend at the waist to the left, and with a strong exhalation through the open mouth, push the arms to the side (Figure D). The breath should be synchronized with the movement, as it is in *sanchin kata*, and should begin and end together. Inhalations accompany the *mawashi uke* movements, while the exhalations are matched with each stretch. Return to the start position, switch hands, and repeat the exercise to the right.

Although found in many *kata* throughout the *Goju ryu* system, and in the *kata* from many other schools of *karate*, the *mawashi uke, tora uchi* (circular block, tiger strike) combination is always connected to a particular breathing pattern: inhaling with the block, and exhaling with the strike. In some *kata*, these actions are performed quickly, while in other *kata* they are performed with a heavy, deliberate feeling. Nevertheless, the combination of physical movement and coordinated breathing is nowhere better felt than during *sanchin kata*. Here, the slow movements and the deep breathing concentrate the sensation of harmony between the physical and the cerebral. Together, this combination often leads to results that amount to more than the sum of its parts.

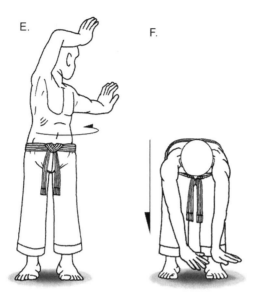

As well as stretching to the sides, a backward (Figure E) and forward (Figure F) stretch is also performed. Always beginning from the same posture (Figure A) and performing *mawashi uke* before moving in the same direction as the arm being held out in front, the backward twist should be done with care taken to keep the body upright as if twisting on a vertical alignment that runs directly through the center of the body.

Arm swings (next page), with the hand formed into a fist, are found in the *Goju ryu kata, saifa,* as well as in the opening sequence of the *Shotokan kata, chinte*. It is yet one more technique that is common to many schools of *karate* and no doubt harks back to a time before individual schools existed. In spite of the often-ingrained ideologies that exist in the minds of many followers of today's *karate* styles, the physical evidence is all around to show how such thinking is fundamentally flawed.

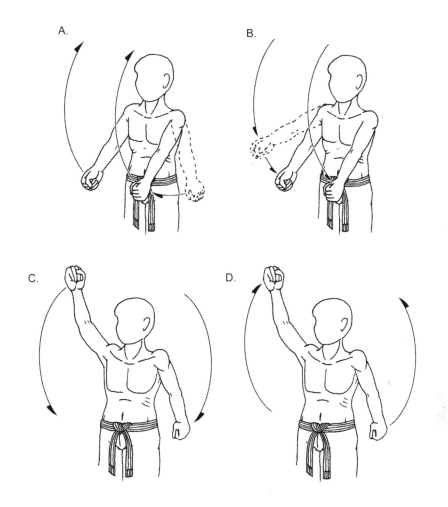

Junbi-Undo 12

Stand naturally and swing the arms backward in a large circular motion (Figure A). Begin slowly and then swing as quickly as possible several times. Reverse the swing (Figure B), remembering to start slowly and end fast.

Finally, swing one arm forward and the other arm backward at the same time (Figure C). Follow the same pattern of slow and quick swings before reversing the direction of each arm (Figure D), swinging each arm in the opposing direction to bring the exercise to a close. Throughout the whole exercise, the arms should be held completely relaxed with no muscle tension at all being used.

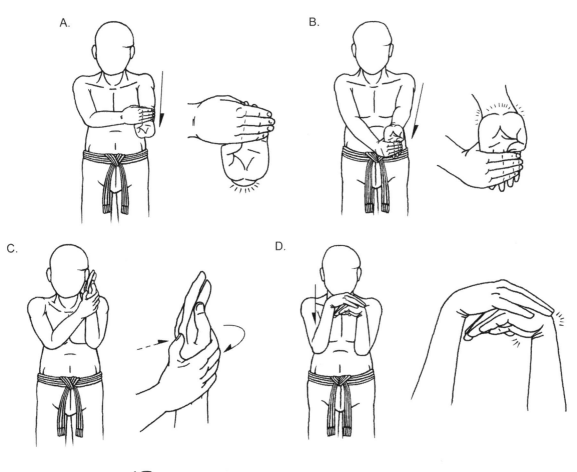

A.

B.

C.

D.

Junbi-Undo 13

Remaining in *heiko dachi* (natural stance), place the left hand on the side of the body with the fingers pointing up (Figure A). The fingers of the right hand cross over the front of the fingers of the left hand. Slowly push the left arm out straight while maintaining contact with the right hand; this push begins to stretch the fingers of the left hand backward. The point of the exercise is to increase the flexibility of the wrist and fingers, while at the same time allow, with the gripping hand, a chance to become accustomed to controlling another person when applying a wrist or finger lock, something that becomes apparent in the final three positions of this exercise.

Return the left hand to the side of the body and rotate it so that the fingers now point downward (Figure B). From here, push the left arm back out again and insert the thumb of the right hand behind the left, placing it firmly in the center of the back of the hand. Apply forward pressure with the thumb on the outstretched hand while pulling the fingers backward. As well as giving the fingers of one hand a good stretch, this position permits the opposite hand to mimic a basic controlling grip.

Release the grip on the fingers, but maintain contact by allowing the thumb of the right hand to keep in touch with the back of the left hand. Bend the left arm at the elbow and bring it up into a *chudan uke* (mid-level blocking position). At the same time swing the fingers of the right hand around the back of the left hand and grab the large thumb muscle (*abductor pollicis brevis*) with the fingers. Keeping the forearm vertical and the joints of the wrist and elbow one above the other (Figure C), apply pressure with the right hand to twist the left hand; pulling the left thumb backward toward the center of the body while the right thumb is pushing in the opposite direction does this.

In the fourth and final part of this exercise, release the grip with the fingers and roll the left hand inward so that the palm is facing down and the fingers are pointing toward the right-hand side of the body. This action should be completed while keeping the hands in contact with each other, first, through the right thumb and then through the palm of the right hand sliding over the top of the left hand. With both elbows pointing down, bring pressure to bear on the back of the left hand (Figure C). The knuckles of the left hand should sit in the center of the right palm. Once again this posture not only stretches the wrist joint, but also mimics the hand position applied when controlling an opponent and reinforces the *karateka*'s introduction to the concept of *muchimi*. When the sequence is complete, repeat the same four parts of this exercise on the opposite side.

Muchimi is a word used in the Okinawan dialect (*hogen*) to describe the texture of rice when it has been pounded into a sticky, glutinous consistency. In *Goju ryu karate*, the word is used to portray a feeling of connection with either the ground, the parts of our own body as when the arms cross each other during blocking, for example, or when contact is made with another person. It is a similar feeling to magnetism, if I can borrow a scientific term. Once contact is made with the other person, you apply your body's weight to keep it there. Once *muchimi* is understood, it allows control of an opponent while alleviating the need to grab onto or hold him.

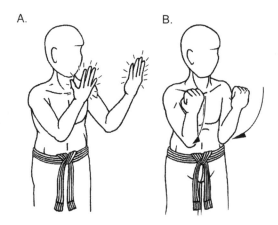

A.   B.

Junbi-Undo 14

Assume a *heiko dachi* (natural stance), making sure the feet are slightly wider than shoulder width and parallel; hold both arms in the *chudan uke* (mid-level block) posture. Without raising your center of gravity or the shoulders, stretch the arms out a little and open the hands and fingers as wide as possible (Figure A), taking in a deep breath through the nose while you do so. Keeping the energy in the fingers, exhale strongly through the open mouth and make a fist with both hands.

Take care to close down the armpit on both sides with the exhalation (Figure B). Keep in mind also that the toes should stretch forward and then grip the floor hard while the hands become fists. Squeeze the abdominal muscles to push the air out and focus on the body's center (*tanden*), exactly as in the *kata sanchin*. Relax back into the original posture and repeat the exercise three times. The relationship between this exercise and the fundamental *kata* of *Goju ryu* is clear, and by its inclusion in the *junbi undo* routine, new students are introduced immediately to the foundations of the *karate* they are about to start learning.

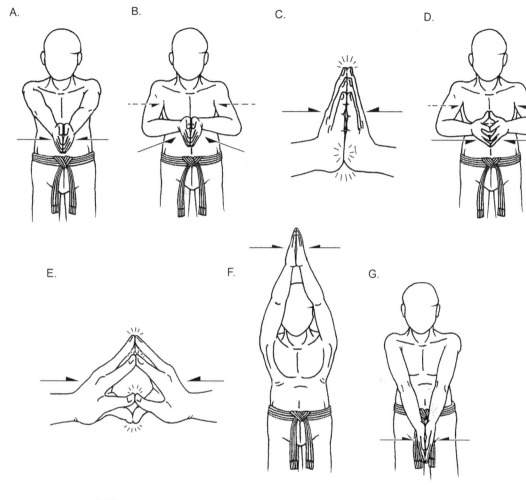

A. B. C. D.

E. F. G.

Junbi-Undo 15

Standing in *heiko dachi*, push the palms of the hands together hard and stretch the arms out in front of the chest (Figure A), inhaling while you do so.

Continue to push the hands together hard while you draw them back toward the chest (Figure B) and exhale through the open mouth.

Making a line between both elbows, try to draw the wrists back a little beyond that line to stretch the wrist joints (Figure C).

Breathe in one more time and while you exhale, focus the pressure on the fingertips (Figures D and E).

This exercise is repeated by stretching above the head (Figure F) and also toward the ground (Figure G). In each case, a strong exhalation accompanies the hands return to the body (Figure B), and care is taken not to raise the shoulders. Each time the hands return to the body, focus pressure on the wrist first and then on the fingertips, as seen in Figures C and E.

In the *Goju ryu kata seipai*, near the beginning, a drop is made into *shiko dachi* (low stance) and from this posture the right elbow is used, either in a striking *(hiji uchi)* action or in a blocking action *(hiji uke)*. Regardless of which action is taken, the block or the strike, the feeling in the arms during the kata is the same as in this exercise.

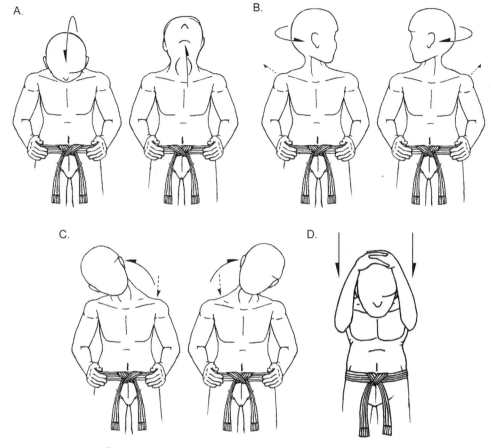

A.

B.

C.

D.

Junbi-Undo 16

Standing in *heiko dachi*, (Figure A), natural stance, with the hands resting on the hips, drop the chin to the chest and breathe in through the nose. Without holding the breath, move the head slowly backward as far as it will go, breathing out through the open mouth while you do so. As always, the physical movement and the breath should be synchronized to begin and end at the same time. Relax the shoulders and focus the mind on the harmony of the breath and posture while the head is gently moved from one position to the next and back again. Several repetitions should be completed.

From a natural position, breathe in through the nose and turn the head to the left, breathing out as you go and making sure the right shoulder is pushing backward to enhance the stretch (Figure B). From there, slowly turn the head to the right, inhaling and exhaling while you complete the move, and remember to now push the left shoulder backward. This exercise should also be repeated several times.

Holding the head naturally (Figure C), breathe in before dropping the head over to one side on an exhalation while pushing the opposite shoulder down toward the ground. Hold this for just a second before moving the head slowly over to the other side.

Keeping the body upright and standing in a natural posture, cup the hands over the back of the head (Figure D). Keep the elbows tucked in and the back up straight; allow the arms to become heavy, gently stretching the top of the spine. Hold this for ten seconds before slowly releasing the pressure from the arms and returning to a natural position.

3 LIFTING TOOLS

I have divided the tools into two groups, those that are gripped and picked up and those that involve various degrees of impact. When training in *hojo undo*, you are free to use any tool in any order; it is not necessary to follow the sequence set out in this book. Neither do all the tools have to be used to gain some benefit from this type of training. If certain equipment proves impossible to construct or find, make the best with what you have. This is how the Okinawans of old approached their training and still do today. Okinawan *karate* is not based on performance statistics measured off against some benchmark figure, but rather on how well you are doing now compared to when you started. *Hojo undo* is as much about gaining confidence through the reality of working with these tools as it is about improving your physical strength.

Makiagi – Wrist Roller

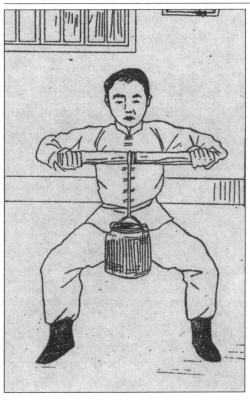

A very difficult way to use the *makiagi* is depicted in this old Chinese drawing.

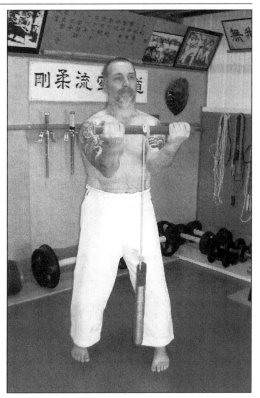

The author (aged 53) training with the *makiagi*, made from old window weights, at his *dojo* in Tasmania.

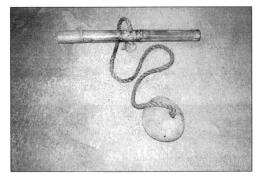

This ancient looking tool was in fact made by Richard Barrett and is used in his private *dojo* in Almeria, Spain.

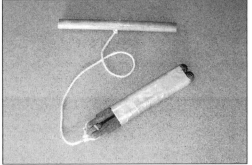

Deceptively simple to look at and easy to make, this tool will test everyone who uses it.

This most basic of tools can be found around the world wherever people gather to develop their bodies. In the earliest versions, rocks were tied with a length of cord or chain to the center of a short piece of wood, and raised and lowered by use of gripping and wrist power alone. During conversations with Tetsuhiro Hokama *sensei*[7] at his *karate* and *kobudo* museum in Nishihara, Okinawa, I discovered there is some consensus among the martial arts community that the weights from ancient looms were among the earliest of the everyday items used in the evolution of this tool, although just as clearly, other workplace items could have been utilized. The heavy stones placed over the thatched roofs to help keep them in place during the typhoon season and the makeshift anchors for the small fishing boats are just two of the other possible candidates for initial inspiration that spring to mind. Over the years, and according to the circumstances of the practitioner, the specifics of any tool may alter. However, the intention remains constant: to push the mind and body hard against the resistance of the tool and see which one wins.

Makiagi Exercises

A. B. C.

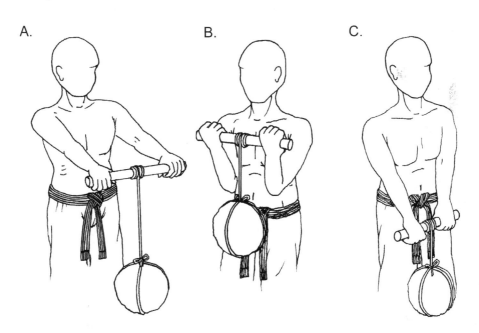

Standing, either naturally or in *sanchin dachi*, with arms outstretched, the palms facing down and the weight of the tool resting on the floor, begin to raise the weight by rolling the rope around the shaft using only the extension and contraction of your grip (Figure A). First using one hand and then the other, try to keep the shaft on an even keel and do not let it wobble up and down while the weight begins to lift. If this happens, it breaks the isolation of the wrist muscles and brings the shoulder muscles into play. The whole idea is to make the fingers and the wrists work hard when lifting and lowering the weight. Keep the head in a natural position, the back straight, and using peripheral vision, watch the weight rise and fall. Once the weight has been raised, reverse the gripping action and return the weight to the ground in the same controlled manner. The action should be smooth and flowing throughout the lift and descent. Although the adoption of a particular stance is not strictly necessary, as long as the back remains upright and not arched, standing in *sanchin dachi* helps link the exercise more closely to *karate* and with the feeling of "fixing" yourself to the ground. Turning the hands over, palms facing up, helps relieve some of the lactic acid build-up in the forearms and allows training to continue.

Bending the arms into the familiar *sanchin* double *chudan uke* posture (Figure B) also gives a different feeling for the exercise. Just remember to keep the shaft moving smoothly and on a level plane and not to lose the isolation of the muscles being targeted.

If these exercises prove to be too difficult, start by holding the arms low (Figure C) and in front of the body. This may well be an appropriate way to start working with the tool for many people, especially those who are slightly built. Regardless of the way in which the tool is being worked, always endeavor to harmonize the breath with the movement of the body and the exercise being done. If the breath is not working with you, it is working against you—there is no neutral ground with this.

Makiagi Construction Notes

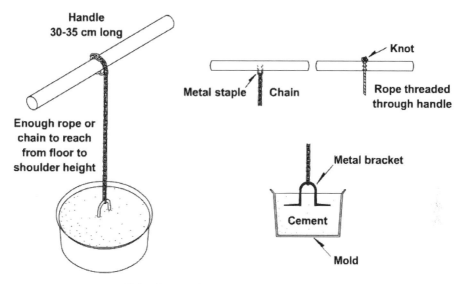

**Handle
30-35 cm long**

**Enough rope or
chain to reach
from floor to
shoulder height**

Metal staple   **Chain**

Knot

**Rope threaded
through handle**

Metal bracket

Cement

Mold

Make the weight to your requirement

A piece of dowel, a length of rope or chain, and a suitable weight make this very effective tool.

You need a rounded piece of wood, fourteen to sixteen inches (30-35 cm) long, a length of rope or chain long enough to stretch from the floor to the height of your shoulders, and a weight that can be made of almost anything. Fix one end of the rope/chain to the weight and the other end to the center of the wooden handle. This is best achieved by drilling a hole through the center of the handle, threading the rope/chain through it first, and then tying it off. The *makiagi* I use weighs 14 lbs. (6.5 kg) and is made from weights once found in the construction of houses as the counterbalance to open and close windows. Each of these iron weights weighs 7 lbs. (3.25 kg), and I have taped two of them together.

Chiishi – Strength Stones

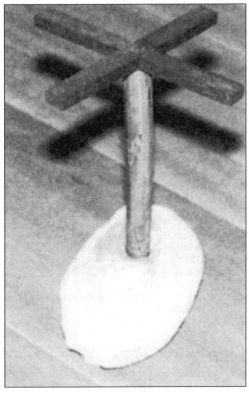

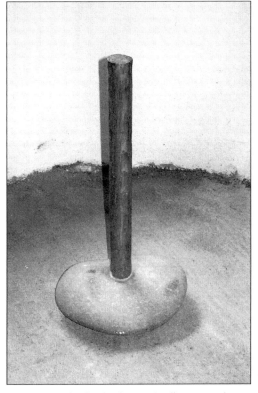

One pre-*karate* use of the *chiishi* can be seen in this example. Here the cross pieces at the top of the handle spin. The implement was used in winding up threads during the manufacture of textiles throughout Okinawa.

Another example of Richard Barrett's adherence to the Okinawan tradition of making tools from resources available. In this case, a length of strong wood and a heavy stone.

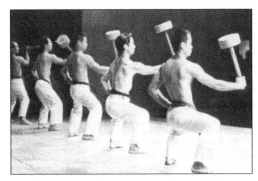

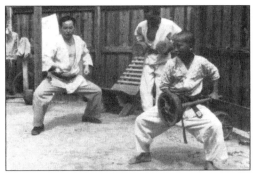

Jundokan students demonstrating with the *chiishi*, October 1973. The demonstration was held to mark the 20th anniversary of Chojun Miyagi's death.

Meitoku Yagi teaching *chiishi* technique in his backyard *dojo* c. 1955. In the background his son, Meitatsu is seen working with home-made barbells.

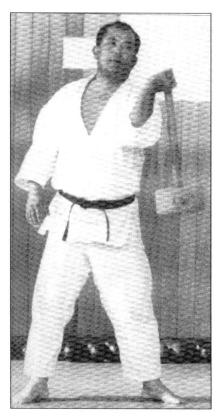

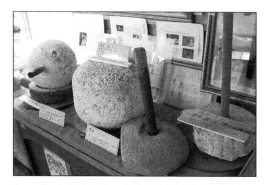

A couple of old *chiishi* on display at the Okinawa Karate Museum in Nishihara. Alongside them, a *sashi ishi* and a twin handle *chiishi*. An excellent display showing some of the diversity behind the single idea of lifting a stone.

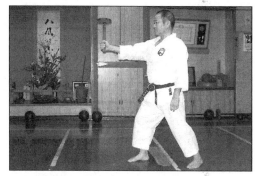

Eiichi Miyazato (1922-1999), the author's teacher. This photo was taken when he was 52 years old in 1973. The founder of the Jundokan *dojo*, after the death of his teacher Chojun Miyagi (1888-1953), he inherited all his teacher's *hojo undo* tools.

Takayoshi Nagamine, son of Shoshin Nagamine and present headmaster of the *Matsubayashi* school of *Shorin ryu karate*, training with the *chiishi* at the Kodokan *dojo* in Kume, Okinawa c. 2005.

Tools similar to the *chiishi* have been used for thousands of years throughout Asia and the Middle East. In particular, wrestlers in India have for centuries used a sophisticated array of tools to build, strengthen, and condition their bodies[8] to ready them for the rigors of the fight. Although many of the exercises and tools differ considerably, the fact that the wrestlers utilized tools in this way at all points to a similarity of thought between them and their Okinawan counterparts. I find it interesting that just as it was the Buddhist monk Bodhidharma[9] who is said to have traveled from India to China in the year A.D. 520, bringing with him the seeds of what would eventually become the fighting techniques of Okinawan *karate*, the Okinawans themselves would also develop a strong belief in the use of tools to supplement their training and condition their bodies.

On Okinawa, the *chiishi* would seem to have originated from the use of two objects in particular: the small grinding stones used in the preparation of food and the looms used as an aid during the spinning process in the production of local textiles.[10] Given the everyday nature of both these activities, either is a likely candidate for the pre-*karate* use of the *chiishi*, thus placing the tool in close proximity to a *karateka* wishing to find something to lift.

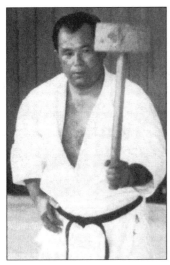

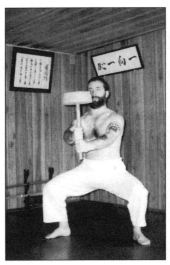

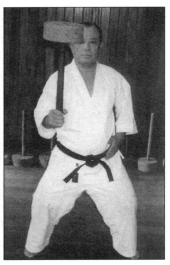

Eiichi Miyazato was not only a *karate* master (10th *Dan*), but a Kodokan judo 8th *Dan* too. He had the rare distinction of having never been thrown in a *judo* competition.

The author, aged 40, training at the original Shinseidokan *dojo*, c. 1995.

Even in old age, Miyazato *sensei* shown at 76 years of age continued to practice *hojo undo*.

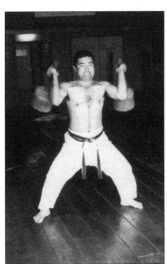

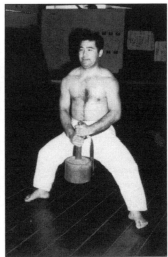

Morio Higaonna working with two *chiishi* at the same time at the Yoyogi *dojo* in Tokyo c. 1970.

During the same workout, he uses a particularly heavy *chiishi* with both hands. Note his impressive shoulder muscle development.

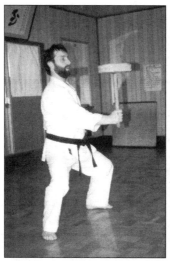
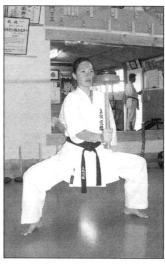

The author training at Morio Higaonna *sensei*'s *dojo* in Kiyose, Tokyo, during the summer of 1987.

Iyn Ang, a female student from Singapore, training at the Shinseidokan *dojo* with a *chiishi* weighing 11 lbs. (5 kg).

Merely by picking up the *chiishi*, you are working the fingers, the wrists, and the arms, and developing, as you do so, stronger muscles with which to grab, choke, poke, or punch an opponent. Having a vise-like grip is a weapon seldom used, developed, or even sought after by many of today's *karateka* because they focus on the acquisition of straight punches and excessively high kicks. As with every other tool, it is important to develop harmony between the body, the breath, and the mind (intention). If one or more of these elements is missing, the connection between the *hojo undo* exercise and *karate* technique is severely hindered, if not lost altogether. There are many exercises that can be done with the *chiishi*, far more than the scope of this book will allow; therefore only three single-grip and three double-grip exercises have been shown. Each one is performed slowly and methodically with the aim of harmonizing the body, breath, and mind in one single action. Even if these were the only exercises used, the tool still promotes strength in the fingers, wrists, arms, shoulders, and back. The repetitive squatting into *shiko dachi* over time helps to develop stronger legs.

Lifting the Chiishi (Single Handle)

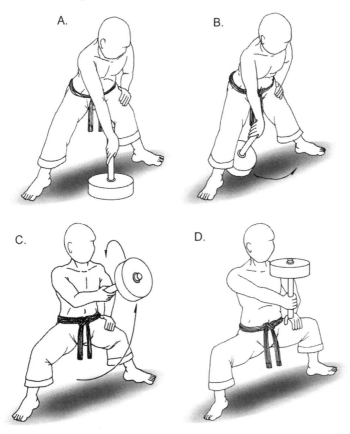

A.

B.

C.

D.

There are a number of ways to lift this tool but the following are two of the most common methods used. The first method is recommended for those who have never worked with this tool before because it makes a less complicated use of gaining momentum to make the lift, though as always, it still requires the *karateka* to develop a "feeling" of harmony with the *chiishi* to prevent it from falling out of control.

In the first method, stand before the tool with your legs open wide enough to drop into *shiko dachi* (Figure A). Grasp the end of the handle with one hand while the other hand rests lightly on the thigh. Then, swing the *chiishi* between the legs to gain momentum (Figure B) before bringing it up in an arc in front of the body (Figure C) and settling down into *shiko dachi*, gripping the ground with the toes while this is done (Figure D). This is the starting position for the most common exercises. As the tool swings upward, inhale and then exhale while the body drops into the stance. Try to keep the posture of the upper body as natural as possible, with the back upright and the arm held out straight. The legs are tensed by pushing the knees backward, and the feet grip the floor when the tool is brought to a halt in front of the body so that the eyes can just see over the top of it.

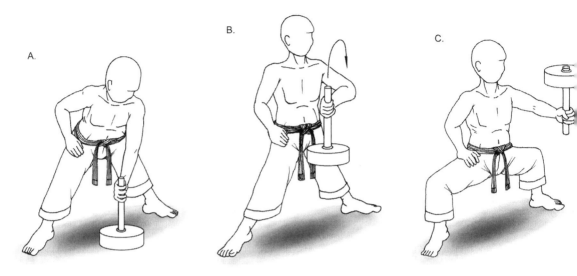

The second method of lifting can be seen at the start of exercise one and requires a little more control of the tool to execute smoothly. The legs and body take up the same starting position as before, but the difference with this lift is in the direction the tool travels and the increased coordination needed between your body and the tool itself. The lifting hand grips the end of the handle while employing a twist along the length of the arm with the palm now facing away from the body (Figure A). Bringing the tool up in as straight a vertical lift as possible, the head of the tool is allowed to carry on upward while the gripping hand is let slip quickly under it (Figure B).

At that point, with the head of the tool above your head height, sit back down into *shiko dachi*, lower the tool, and assume the starting position prior to exercising (Figure C). As before, the upward lift is accompanied by an inhalation, while the exhalation is matched with the downward action of the arm and the legs settling back into *shiko dachi*. The eyes are looking forward, just over the top of the tool.

An alternative way of holding the tool, if the weight of the *chiishi* is a little too heavy, is to grip further along the handle toward the weight. This grip eases the pressure on the wrists and allows the tool to be used. However, care should be exercised if adopting this grip to avoid being struck by the protruding end of the handle.

Single-Handle Chiishi

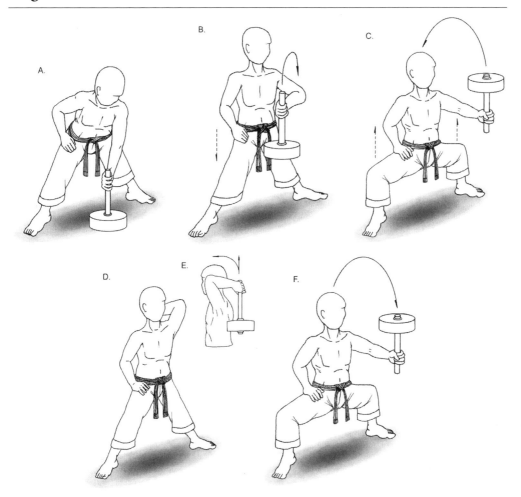

A. B. C.

D. E. F.

Exercise 1

From the starting position (Figure C), lift the tool in a chopping action over the shoulder while you straighten the legs and stand up (Figure D); let the *chiishi* drop behind the shoulder, relaxing (Figure E) the muscles of the arm while maintaining a tight grip. Take a deep breath in through the nose before breathing out through the mouth and sitting back into *shiko dachi*; when you do so, engage the tricep muscles at the back of the upper arm to lift the tool clear of the shoulder and then, in a chopping action, bring it back over the shoulder before coming to a halt in the starting position (Figure F). This exercise (minus the lift) should be repeated at least ten times before returning the *chiishi* to the floor and commencing the same exercise with the opposite arm.

With all lifts, take care to grip the handle firmly, squeeze the fingers tightly, keep the tool under control, and keep the back upright and straight. This may prove difficult at first but with patience and a *chiishi* that is not too heavy, progress can be made fairly quickly. Be sure to close the armpit at the end of each exercise to connect the entire body with the tool. An open or relaxed armpit disconnects the arm from the body and leaves the muscles of the latter on their own to deal with the weight of the tool. The open armpit shortens the number of times the tool can be worked due to the early onset of fatigue. This exercise is particularly good for developing strength in the upper arms as well as the shoulders. Of course, every exercise done with the *chiishi* leads to improved strength in the hands and wrists.

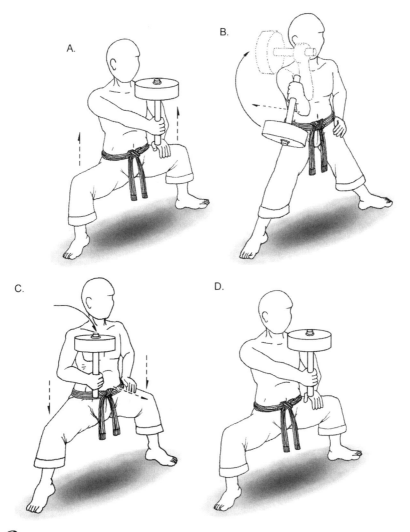

A.

B.

C.

D.

Exercise 2

This time, stand up from the starting position (Figure A), and let the *chiishi* roll backward over the shoulder (Figure B). You should reach the upright position at the same time as the tool arrives at the side of the body (Figure C). All this is done when breathing in. The elbow is tucked back and the armpit closed, similar to a chambered arm in a punching position. Without stopping, and keeping a rhythmical action, drop down slowly into *shiko dachi* while the *chiishi* is pushed straight out to the front, exhaling with the drop (Figure D). The movement and the breath should stop at exactly the same time, and the exercise can be repeated again from this posture, building as you go the number of repetitions in accordance with your strength. The rolling action of this exercise is of particular benefit to the muscles of the upper arm.

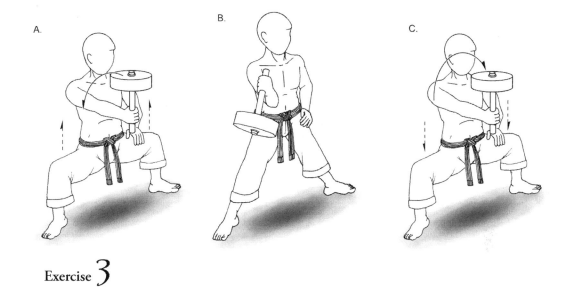

A.

B.

C.

Exercise 3

With this, the last of these basic single-grip exercises, the focus is on the wrist and forearm. From the starting posture in *shiko dachi* (Figure A), stand up slowly and inhale, allowing the *chiishi* to roll to the outside, resulting in an arm position not unlike that found in *chudan uke* (Figure B). Then, simply reverse the movement and sit back down into *shiko dachi* while exhaling (Figure C). Remember to keep the wrist strong by gripping the tool as tightly as possible with the fingers. Keep the *chiishi* moving as if rolling on an invisible surface just in front of you and do not let it drop back behind the wrist, because this alters the stress put on the arm and joints. The synchronization of the breath with the lifting and dropping of the body, over time, results in a heightened sense of harmony between breath and body movement, and this in turn enhances the fighting techniques of your *karate*.

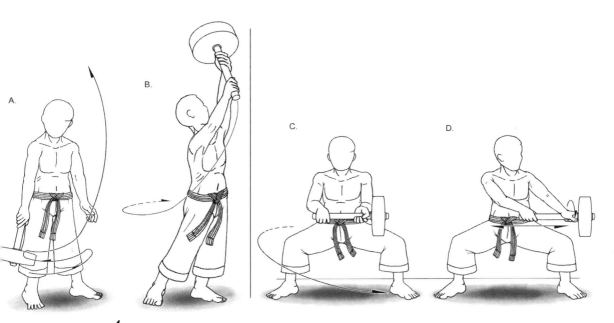

Exercise 4

Begin by holding the *chiishi* in the right hand while standing with the right leg forward. From here swing the tool back and forth to gain some momentum (Figure A); two or three swings are sufficient before lifting the tool high above the head as illustrated (Figure B). At this point draw a deep breath in while stepping sharply forward (edge on), dropping into *shiko dachi* when you do so and bring the *chiishi* to the position shown (Figure C) in front of the body. From here, three short, sharp, stabbing movements are made over the course of one exhalation. With each outward thrust, the arms are extended and twisted in a similar way to the twist put into the end of a regular *karate* punch (Figure D). On the return, the twist is reversed. After the third movement, simply stand up, step backward, and assume the original position. During this time the breathing returns to its normal rhythm. Repeat at least six times before swapping over and doing the exercise with the left arm.

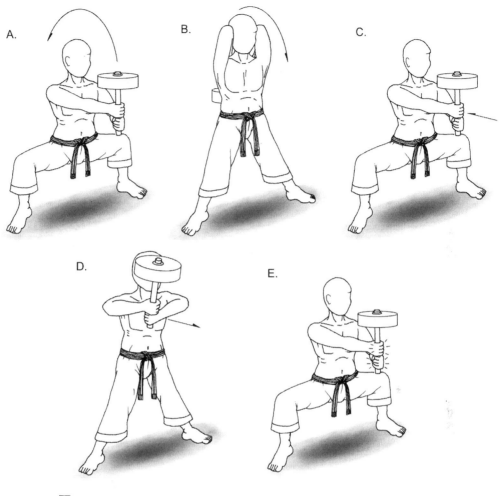

Exercise 5

Using both hands to grip the tool, place the left hand at the end of the handle and the right hand next to it. Then, in the same fashion as the first single-handed lift, raise the tool into the starting position (Figure A). From there, execute a simple chopping action, breathing in while the *chiishi* is lifted behind the back (Figure B) and exhale while the body drops slowly back down into *shiko dachi* (Figure C). Immediately raise the body up once more, only this time loosening the grip a little, allowing the arms to bend (Figure D). Re-tighten the grip and sit back into *shiko dachi* while the tool is pushed forward once again, but now as if wringing out a wet towel (Figure E). This action is accompanied with a strong exhalation. Both the breath and the body movements should remain synchronized throughout. To gain maximum benefit from this exercise, return the tool to the ground after each lift and change the grip over, remembering to maintain a sense of rhythm as you do so.

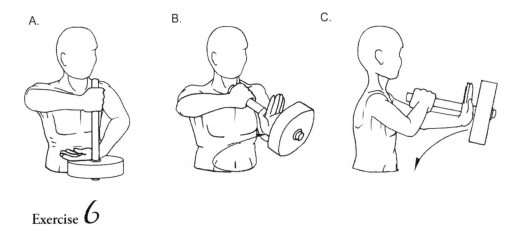

A.   B.   C.

Exercise 6

Standing in *sanchin dachi*, hold the end of the handle with the right hand in the grip shown in Figure A. The left hand is placed toward the head of the tool with the palm facing upward. From there execute a *hikei uke* (open-handed grasping block) action, rotating the hand while the block develops (Figure B). The right hand allows the *chiishi* to move with the block but should not be used to lift it, because this takes away some of the resistance the blocking arm is working against and lessens the benefit of the exercise. An inward breath accompanies the first half of the block, while pushing the tool upward and outward (Figure C). The exhalation begins when the blocking hand returns to the body and the starting position (Figure A).

By using these and other exercises, and with a well-constructed *chiishi* that is heavy enough to offer a challenge, you will steadily develop greater strength in the hands, arms, and legs. Those new to the *chiishi* should consider using a lightweight tool until they have learned to use it safely and only then moving on to a heavier one.

Chiishi (Single Handle) Construction Notes

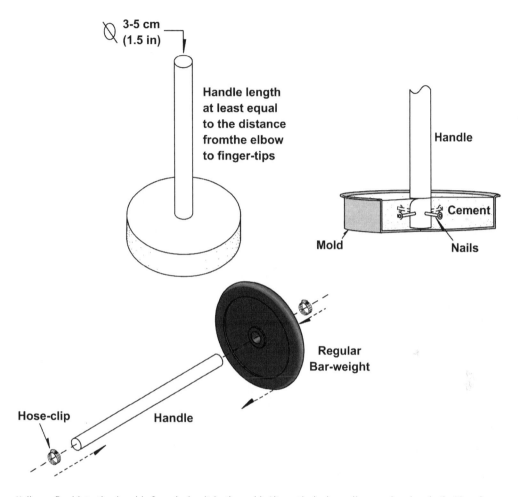

3-5 cm (1.5 in)

Handle length at least equal to the distance from the elbow to finger-tips

Handle

Mold

Cement

Nails

Hose-clip

Handle

Regular Bar-weight

Nails are fixed into the dowel before placing it in the mold. Alternatively, hose clips are placed on both sides of a regular weight.

You need a length of wood that is at least equal to the distance from the elbow to the tips of the fingers, with a diameter of approximately one and one-half inches (3.5 cm). The weight is made from cement poured into a mold and the handle placed in the center. Care should be taken to keep the handle straight while the cement hardens. To add to the grip of the handle in the cement, nails should be driven through the end of the handle in opposing directions before the handle is placed in the wet cement and left to dry. The *chiishi* I use in my *dojo* weighs 14 lbs. (6.35 kg).

Double-Handle Chiishi

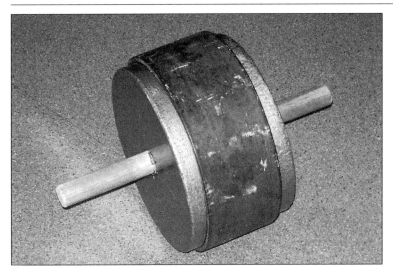

Author's *Chiishi*.

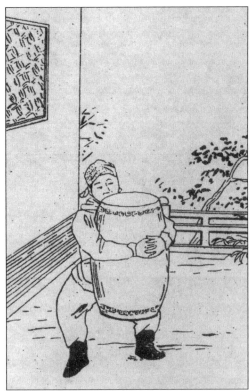

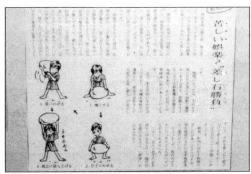

Sashi ishi training advice on display at the Karate Museum in Nishihara. Once a handle was added, the tool was used differently.

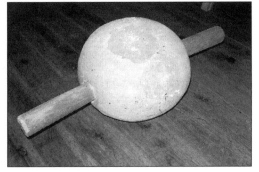

The twin-handle *chiishi* evolved from simply lifting heavy rocks and containers, as seen in this drawing from an ancient Chinese training manual, into the specific lifts done with the tool today.

The twin-handle *chiishi* at the Jundokan in Okinawa.

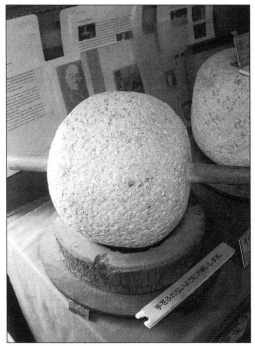

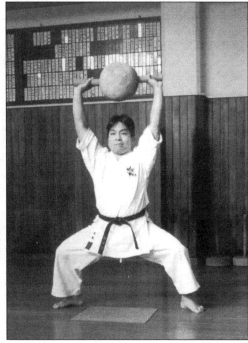

A close-up of the hybrid tool. This one is on display at the Okinawa Karate Museum and shows the merging of two tools leading to the evolution of a third.

A test of timing, strength, and nerve for Satoshi Taba at the Jundokan, Okinawa.

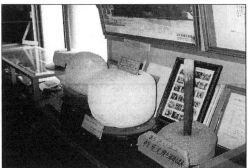

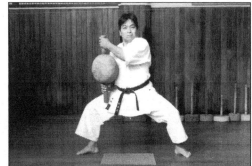

Examples of chiishi at the Okinawa Karate Museum.

Satoshi Taba of the Jundokan *dojo*, Okinawa, training with the twin-handle *chiishi*.

As well as the more common single-handle *chiishi* used by *karateka* on Okinawa and around the world, there exists another *chiishi*, a much heavier one that is used exclusively for two-handed exercises. Less common these days than its single-handled cousin, it affords those *karateka* who use it an opportunity to work their bodies in ways not possible with the more common tool. The following three exercises should be done with even greater care than usual because the weight involved is significantly heavier. Certainly in the early stages, it is advisable to work with a partner when lifting this and the *kongoken*.

The double-handle *chiishi* began life as nothing more than a large rock, weighing

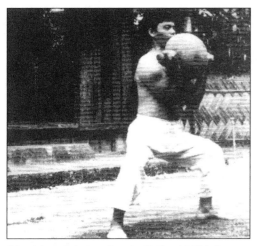

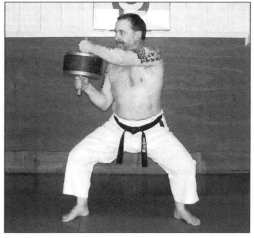

A Jundokan student works out with the *chiishi* during a summer *gasshuku* in Okinawa.

The author training with the *chiishi* at his Shinseidokan *dojo*, Tasmania c. 2008.

around 50 lbs. (23 kg), with the original exercise consisting of little more than picking it up and walking around with it, or lifting it up onto one shoulder before passing it over your head and returning it to the ground on the other side. Eventually, people's favorite rocks were kept and later fashioned into smooth rounded stones (*sashi ishi*) that, in due course, had holes drilled in them and wooden handles inserted through the center. This allowed for a variety of lifting exercises, some of which more closely resembled the moves found in *karate*, and thus targeted the same muscle groups used by *karateka* when training in their fighting art. The benefits from this approach are obvious: a stronger body made for techniques that are more powerful. With the natural physique of the Okinawan male being, until fairly recently, short but sturdy, it comes as no surprise that there has always been a desire among the island's *karate* men to develop their bodies. Many of the great masters of the past employed the concept of *hojo undo* in their daily training.

Anko Azato, for example, was known to have had *hojo undo* tools in various parts of his home. In the book *Tanpenshu: Untold Stories of Gichin Funakoshi*, coauthored by Patrick and Yuriko McCarthy, translated and published 2004 in Brisbane, Australia, Funakoshi relates a story about his teacher, Yatsutsune (Anko) Azato:

> *During my teacher's youth, few martial arts enthusiast could even afford the supplementary training equipment which is commonly associated with training these days. However, Azato was an exception and it was because he was from a family of wealth and position that he could afford such things. In fact, his home looked like one big training facility. Both standing and hanging makiwara were located in various rooms of the Azato residence, along with other training equipment, which included wooden cudgels, stone weights, iron balls for grip strength development, shield and machete, flails, iron truncheons (sai), and even a wooden horse for mounting practice and archery spotting. Master Azato had created a living environment where he could train anytime and anywhere he liked.* (p. 46)

When reading this description for the first time, I could not help but wonder if the stone weights being referred to here were in fact *chiishi*. In 1987, when I was training in Tokyo at the *dojo* of Morio Higaonna, I had the opportunity to visit his home in the outlying district of Kiyose a number of times. His backyard was easily distinguishable from those of his neighbors by the fierce looking *makiwara* planted firmly in the earth, and by the *chiishi* and *kongoken* that stood close by. Inside his home, he had a sheet of A4-sized paper suspended at head height in the doorway to the kitchen, and on it was a crude drawing of a face. The eyes had been cut out to give it the appearance of a grotesque mask. Whenever Higaonna *sensei* walked past it, he would throw out a lightning fast finger strike into one or other of the open eyes. Sometimes he would open the index and middle fingers of his hand and poke them through both eyeholes with the one strike. He told me that if he did it right he could hit the target without tearing the flimsy paper, but if he got it wrong, he would rip the paper and then have to construct another one. In all the visits I made to his home, I only ever saw the one mask.

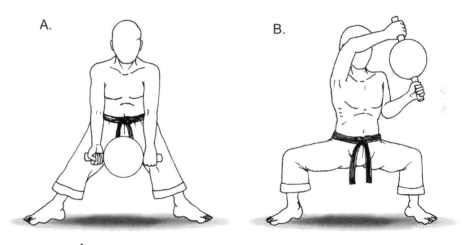

EXERCISE 1

Keeping the back straight and using the legs to lift the *chiishi*, grip the handle (as shown in Figure A) with the right hand palm out, the left hand palm inward; then stand up. From there inhale before dropping quickly into *shiko dachi* (low stance) and throwing the *chiishi* up and out to the side on an exhalation (Figure B). Hold that posture for one or two seconds before returning to the start position and repeating the exercise. Reverse the grip before working the opposite side of the body. In both cases, make sure the legs are locked into a good stance throughout and the head is held in a natural posture, with eyes looking at the *chiishi*.

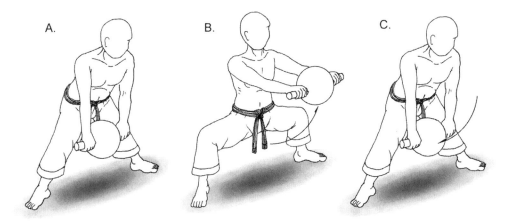

A.   B.   C.

EXERCISE *2*

Both hands grip the *chiishi* with the palms facing inward; from here swing the tool between the legs, which should be straight to gain momentum (Figure A). One swing suffices. Then bring the *chiishi* up and hold it for a brief moment directly out in front of the body while dropping into *shiko dachi* at the same time (Figure B) before letting the tool swing back down (Figure C). The breath should be inhaled through the nose while the swing lifts the tool and exhaled sharply through the open mouth when the tool comes to a stop in front of the body. Because this kind of *chiishi* is traditionally much heavier than its single-handled cousin, the number of repetitions is fewer. Still, every effort should be made to make the number of exercises sufficient to work the body and mind hard. Again, allow the eyes to follow the *chiishi*.

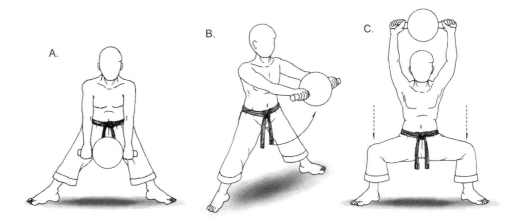

Exercise 3

This exercise is an extension of the previous one. This time, however, the *chiishi* is swung completely vertically and the arms are locked into position directly above the head, while at the same time the body drops down into *shiko dachi* (Figure A). Again, great care should be taken to lock both the legs and the arms into position, while simultaneously using the breath in coordination with the physical movement. The hands should grasp the handle firmly, with the head held naturally and eyes looking forward. Hold this position only for a second before swinging it back in front of the body, between the legs and back up again. In all, this should be done at least three times before placing the tool on the floor and resting. During the lift, an inhalation accompanies the swinging of the *chiishi* upward, and the exhalation is issued when the tool is held above the head and you have dropped into *shiko dachi*.

As with all the tools, a poorly constructed *chiishi* can cause more harm than good. Due to the heavy weight and the nature of the exercises, a poor method of practice with this tool has the potential for very serious injury. Therefore, you should use caution and common sense always, train with a partner, and check every tool, every time, before use, to make sure it is safe. Above all, remember to work with weights that can be controlled.

Chiishi (Double Handle) Construction Notes

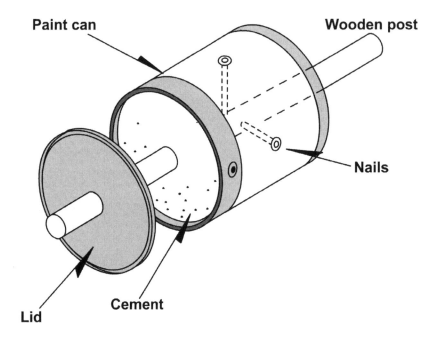

Paint can **Wooden post**

Nails

Cement

Lid

An old paint can filled with cement, with wooden dowel passing through it. Nails are driven into the dowel before inserting it in the can and pouring the cement.

If a large enough stone cannot be found, then make a hole in the bottom of a big old paint can and also through the center of the lid. Place a strong length of wood through both holes and fill the empty can with cement. Do not make the holes too big; the handle should only just pass through them. Replace the lid back on the can, making sure the handle sticks out equally at either end, and allow it to dry. A few nails knocked into the center of the wooden handle before the cement is poured helps stabilize the tool when in use.

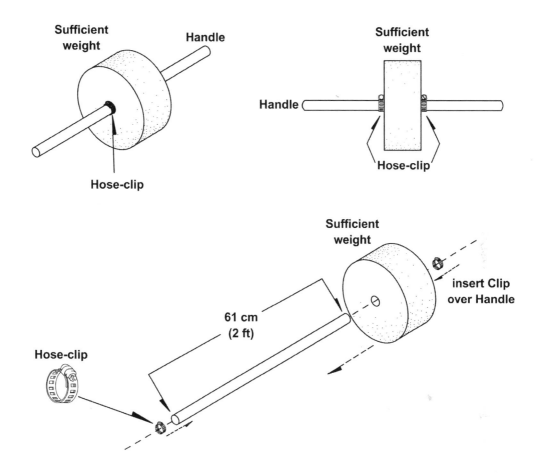

Standard weights require hose clips to be secured on each side.

If the previous method of construction seems too ambitious, then simply purchase enough standard weights to offer sufficient resistance and a length of strong wood with a diameter thick enough to pass tightly through the center hole, to form a handle. Make the handle approximately two feet (61 cm) long. Place it through the center of the weights and secure firmly with nails and hose clips with screws. The *chiishi* I use in my *dojo* weighs almost 50 lbs. (23 kg). It is made from an old flywheel from a tractor and weighs approximately 10 lbs. (4.5 kg), along with two 20 lb. (9 kg) weights.

Nigiri Gami – Gripping Jars

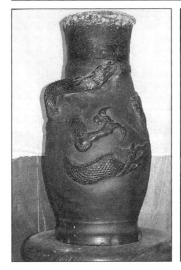

A 200-year-old jar from China on display at the Okinawa Karate Museum in Nishihara.

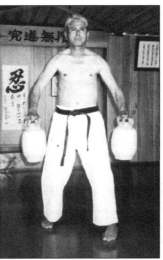

Kosuke Yonamine, Hanshi 9th *Dan Shohei ryu* (*Uechi ryu*) *karate*, training at the author's Shinseidokan *dojo* in Perth, Western Australia in 1997.

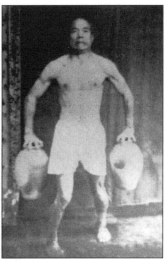

Seiyu Nakasone (1893-1983) of the *Tomari-te* school of *karate*. Note how people used to dress for *karate* training in Okinawa before adopting the now universally worn Japanese *karate-gi*.

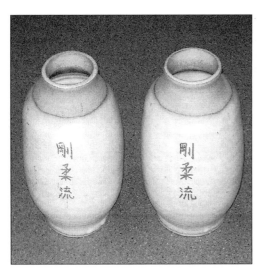

These jars are the oldest of several sets at the author's Shinseidokan. They were made by hand in 1985.

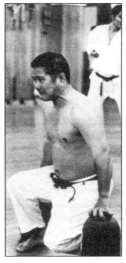

Ko Uehara, today one of Okinawa's leading teachers of *Goju ryu*, seen here as a student at the Jundokan *dojo*, preparing to lift a set of *nigiri game* in 1973.

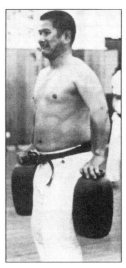

Ko Uehara working with the *nigiri gami* at the Jundokan *dojo*, Okinawa in 1973.

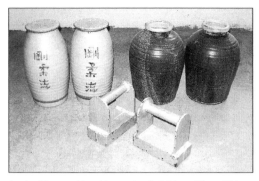

A set of iron *sashi* and two sets of *nigiri gami* from Richard Barrett's private *dojo* in Spain. Note the jars have been filled to the top with cement.

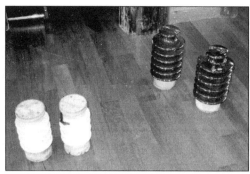

Old power line insulators are also used as *nigiri gami* at Tetsuhiro Hokama *sensei*'s *dojo* in Nishihara, Okinawa.

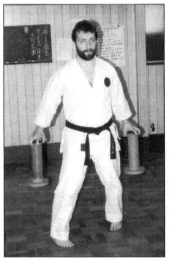

The author training at Morio Higaonna's *dojo* in Kiyose, Tokyo in 1987 with a set of *gami* made from steel pipe.

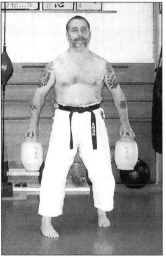

The author during one of his solitary early morning training sessions at his Shinseidokan *dojo*, Tasmania, 2008.

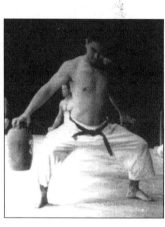

A Jundokan student demonstrates how to use the *nigiri gami* during a demonstration in Naha, October 1973.

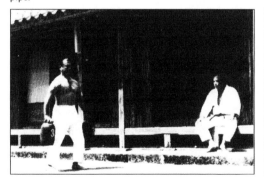

Eiichi Miyazato overseeing *nigiri gami* training during a summer *gasshuku* in Okinawa.

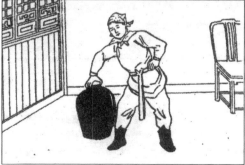

A single-handle lift with a large jar is depicted in this drawing from an old Chinese text.

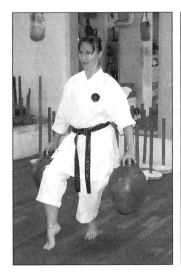 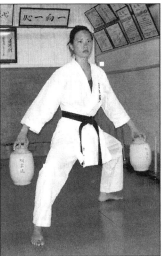 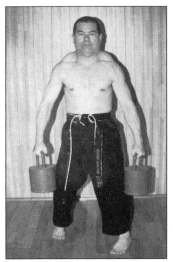

Anni Moynihan of New Zealand, a student at the Higaonna *dojo* in Naha, Okinawa, training both her grip and her stances.

Iyn Ang, a student of the Shinseido-kan *dojo* from Singapore, training her *shiko dachi* stance while strengthening her grip.

Note the shoulder muscle development on this Okinawan *karateka*. His *nigiri gami* resemble Russian kettle bells more than jars. But we must remember to use what we have and make the most of it.

You do not have to look too far to see that this training aid was an object found in almost every household kitchen, shop, or location where things needed to be stored. The history of ceramics on Okinawa is once again linked to China through a long trading history with their giant neighbor. The Tsuboya district of Naha is where many of the Chinese and indigenous artisans set up shop, and even today it remains a cultural oasis amid the hustle and bustle that is modern Naha. Included in the island's tradition for making pots and items of every sort from clay, Okinawan society has a long and illustrious history producing large jars used to house the remains of the dead before being placed in one of the huge turtle-back tombs found dotted on hillsides throughout the island and the rest of the Ryukyu archipelago. Although the gravesites have shrunken in size these days, the ritual of washing the bones of the dead once a year on the day of *Tanabata* (visiting the grave to honor ancestral spirits) for three years following the death is still alive. Thus, the production of large jars can still be found. These days jars are also made specifically for the many *karateka*, indigenous and foreign, who practice with them.

The Nigiri Gami Grip

Used to promote a powerful grip, the jars are held by the fingers in a particular way (as shown) and great care should be taken to master this grip. If the jars are allowed to simply hang by the fingertips, most of the benefits of "gripping" are lost when the resistance transfers to the arm muscles. First of all, it is important to use jars that have the correct size opening for your hands. If the opening is too large, the hands are stretched too far and the proper gripping action cannot be made. Similarly, if the neck of the jar is too small, the hand also fails to hold the tool properly. To hold the jars in the correct manner, the fingertips should be placed evenly around the front of the rim, while the thumb is bent and the edge between the tip and the first joint is pushed hard against the back of the rim. The fingers and the thumb are then squeezed together to hold the jars when lifted from the ground. This method of holding the jars ensures they do not merely hang in the hands. If the jars selected are too heavy, it may prove impossible to lift them using this grip. Therefore, jars that are somewhat light are preferable to start with. As the tool becomes easier to use, sand or stones can be added to the jars to increase their weight. On my first visit to Okinawa in January 1984, I tried to lift the *nigiri gami* at the Higaonna *dojo* in Naha and failed. It took many attempts over three days before I was able to do even the most basic of exercises with them. So persevere and be content to make progress at a steady pace.

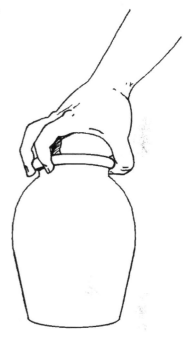

The Nigiri Gami Lift

To lift the jars, it is of course possible to just bend the knees and pick them up. However, when practicing *sanchin kata* with the *nigiri gami*, there is a more formal way to take them from the ground.

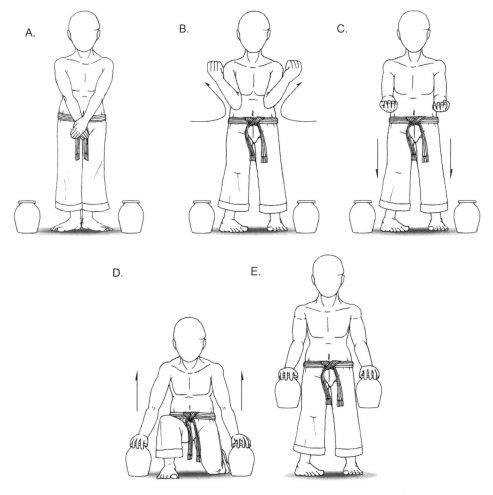

A.

B.

C.

D.

E.

Standing in the *yoi* (get ready) position, just to the left and rear of the jars (Figure A), step out with the right leg and adopt the *sanchin dachi* between them (Figure B). Draw the elbows back (Figure C) and with an inhalation rotate the now open hands until the palms are pointing to the floor. From here, the breath becomes an exhalation when the body squats down (Figure D) allowing the hands to grip the jars. Take the time to make a proper grip at this point because it must last for the length of the *kata*. If necessary, breathe normally while the grip is set, but remember, the aim is to produce smooth, flowing movements with the body and breath acting in harmony. Learn to establish a proper grip quickly.

When ready, take a deep breath in and then stand up (Figure E), exhaling while the body rises and settles back into the *sanchin dachi* before taking the first step forward. It should be noted that none of the striking, trapping, or blocking techniques found in the *sanchin kata* are addressed while holding the jars. Rather, attention is focused on correct breathing, body posture, and the synchronization of each with the other.

Basic Nigiri Gami Exercises

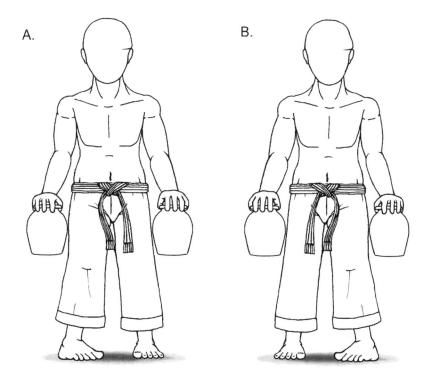

The most common way of using the *nigiri gami* is to walk, using *sanchin dachi* (Figures A and B) while holding the jars at the side and slightly to the rear of the body. Though simple looking at first, the posture requires some effort to get right. The fingers should always face forward with the thumb at the back of the jar. The arm is bent a little and the shoulders should be rolled forward, taking care not to lift them. The idea is to adopt a similar position with regard to the shoulders such as that found during *sanchin kata*. The chest is therefore small, and the back of the shoulders broad. From here, you can simply follow the *embusen* (pattern of steps taken in a *kata*) of *sanchin kata*, or take a less formal approach by moving in a slow and rhythmical fashion, walking forward. After a number of steps, you can simply reverse the stepping and move backward across the floor.

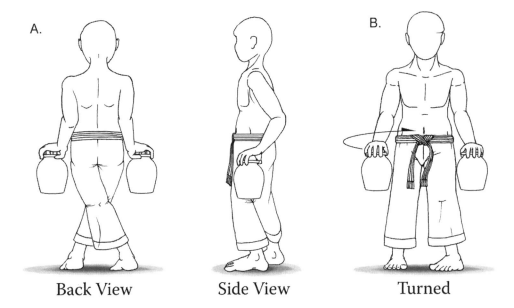

A.

B.

| Back View | Side View | Turned |

At some point, you can introduce a 180-degree turn, and for this the same method of turning found in *sanchin kata* is employed. Keeping the back straight and always stepping across with the right leg in front of the left, plant the sole (*teisoku*) of the right foot down on the floor and allow your body weight to shift into the center (Figure A). From here, twist the hips 180 degrees and assume *sanchin dachi* (Figure B). Make sure the hips are the last thing to turn and that the shoulders and hips are kept in line with each other. Do this by keeping the back upright.

The breathing may differ slightly depending on the expertise of the *karateka* or on the focus being brought to bear on the breath itself. Most beginners with this tool take a step first then breathe in and out using their abdomen to breathe in through the nose and then out through the mouth. The next step is then taken, followed by the next complete breath. The more advanced *karateka* is able to inhale while stepping and begins to exhale the instant the next stance has been established. This second method leads to a more rhythmical and, therefore, more harmonious blending of the breath and the movement. This, in turn, results in a deeper sense of using your whole self—mind, body, and breath—to achieve your intention, and this is a fundamental concept found in all traditional martial arts training. Regardless of which breathing method is used, each movement should be performed with a steady, almost heavy feeling. Good contact with the floor and a feeling of *muchimi* should be maintained throughout all the exercises, even when using different stances such as *nekoashi dachi* (cat stance) and *shiko dachi* (low stance).

Another exercise you can do is to stand in *sanchin dachi* (hourglass stance) and hold a single jar in the palms of the hands close to the chest (Figure A). From there, breathe in through the nose before sliding quickly forward using *suri ashi*. Immediately, when the new position is fixed, squeeze the abdominal muscles, bringing your focus on the *hara* and thrusting the arms out straight while you exhale through the mouth (Figure B). Take care to keep the armpits closed, as in *sanchin kata*,

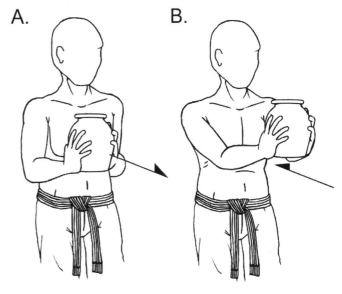

and make sure the outward breath and the thrusting arms are working in harmony. When this move has been completed, reverse it by pushing backward, and on an inward breath, draw the jar back toward the chest. Keep the backward and forward movements in harmony with the inward and outward breaths and do not rush. The idea is to develop a good feeling for your connection to the ground and the synchronization of the breath and the technique, which in this case is the thrust and pull of the arms immediately after a new stance has been made.

Suri ashi is a particular form of *tai sabaki* (body shifting), where a feeling of pushing with one leg and immediately pulling with the other to change your position in relation to an opponent is used. This method of movement is first seen in the *Goju ryu kata*, *gekisai dai ni*, and then used again in *saifa*, *seipai*, *kururunfa*, *seisan*, and *suparinpei*.

The *hara* is a place in the body believed to be its center. By placing two fingers together and laying them at the bottom of your navel, it is possible to find its mystical location. However, you will not find a person's *hara* on any Western medical chart. In Asian martial arts of all kinds, the *hara*, also referred to sometimes as the *tanden* in Japanese or *tan-tien* in Chinese, is the place where *ki* (Japanese) or *chi* (Chinese) is developed. It is the center of your gravity and balance. In *karate* there is a saying: "Develop your *tanden*." On a deeper level, this is pointing to the development of the 'self'.

Nigiri Gami Construction Notes

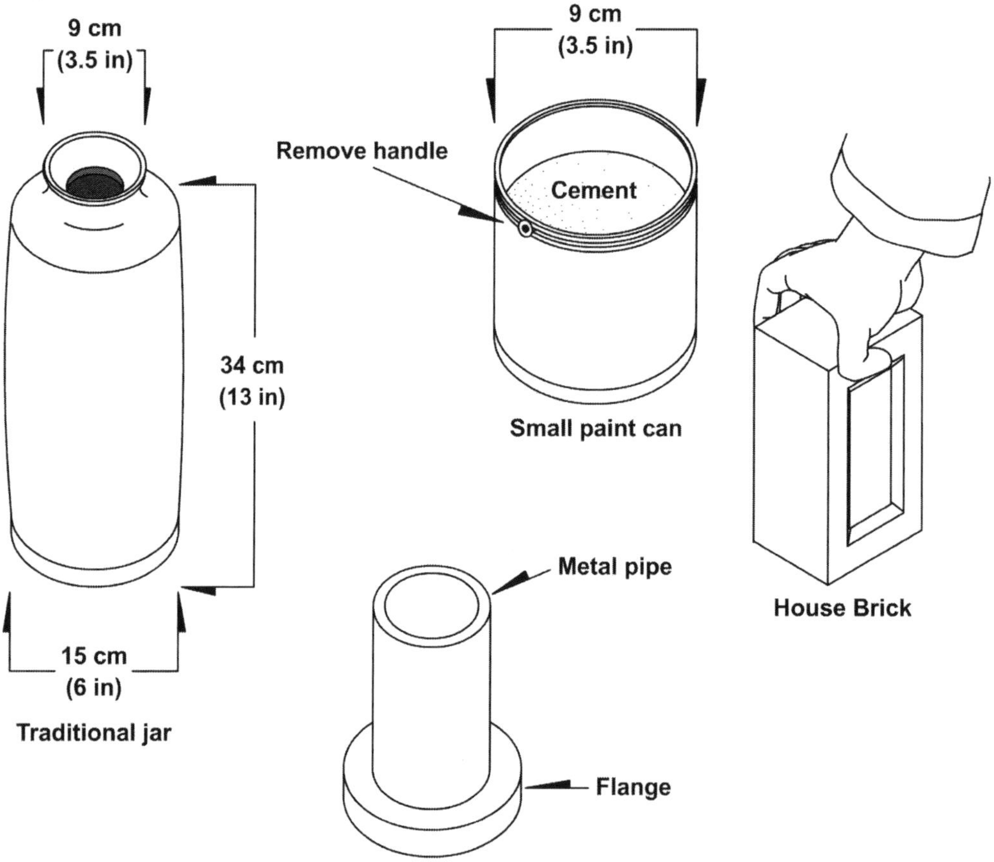

9 cm (3.5 in)

9 cm (3.5 in)

Remove handle

Cement

34 cm (13 in)

Small paint can

Metal pipe

House Brick

15 cm (6 in)

Traditional jar

Flange

House bricks, lengths of pipe, and other items can be used instead of jars.

If it is not possible to find actual jars, you can still train the fingers, wrists, arms, and shoulders in this way, by utilizing other things, such as common house bricks, old cans, or lengths of steel pipe with the appropriate diameter to allow the correct grip. Like many other methods of training in *hojo undo*, our own imagination is often the key to finding ways that augment our martial art and promote a strong mind and healthy body. The jars I use weigh 12 lbs. each (5 kg).

Tan – Barbell

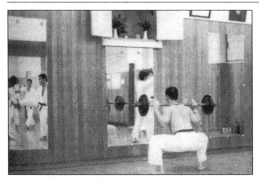

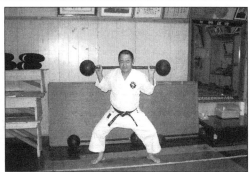

Here a student of the Jundokan *dojo* in Okinawa is using a modern barbell like a *tan* to help strengthen his legs. *Tan* and barbells have always been interchangeable, using whichever comes to hand. This photograph was taken in 1973.

Takayoshi Nagamine, headmaster of the *Matsubayashi* school of *Shorin ryu karate*, using the *tan* to offer resistance while working his legs doing squats, during training at his Kodokan *dojo* in Kume, Okinawa, in 2006.

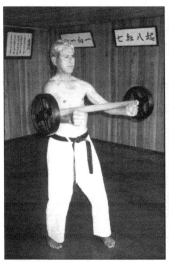

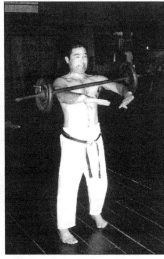

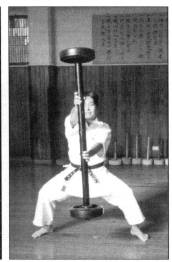

Kosuke Yonamine training with the *tan* at the author's Shinseidokan *dojo* in Perth, Western Australia, in 1998.

Morio Higaonna using a modern barbell as a *tan* at his Yoyogi *dojo* in Tokyo in 1973.

Satoshi Taba of the Jundokan *dojo*, making it look easy.

The *tan* is perhaps one of the more immediately recognizable tools to the Western eye, its shape and form being so close to the modern barbell found in gymnasiums the world over. However, the range of exercises using the *tan* differs greatly from the kind of lifting generally associated with the Western barbell. This is not to suggest that one method of training is in any way superior or more insightful than the other when it comes to building the body's strength and ability to withstand impact; rather, the exercises involving the *tan* are pointed more directly toward the techniques and postures found in *karate* practice.

Two large stones, a length of rope, and a shaft of strong wood were all that was needed to construct the early versions of the *tan*. Later, with the arrival of railways and mechanized farming equipment in China and Okinawa, iron wheels of different sizes and weights became more common. Cement, too, poured into molds made from buckets on either end of a stout post and allowed to set were also used. Regardless of the material employed, the basic concepts remain the same today as they have always been—use whatever materials are at hand, build with caution, and use with care. What follows are five of the many different exercises that can be done with this tool, each one targeting a different part of the body. It is important to remember however, that *karate* requires that your whole body be used in the execution of technique. *Hojo undo* is no different in this regard and the breath, the body, and the mind must all play their part in the working of each tool. To do otherwise is to invite accident or injury.

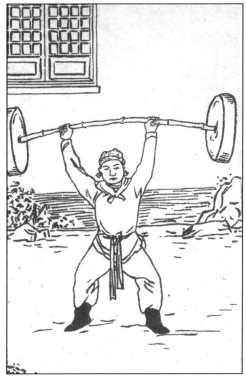

The *tan* in use, as illustrated in an old Chinese manual on martial arts.

I acknowledge that these days science is often adopted to bolster the modern approach to all things physical. Despite this, my approach is not to educate *karateka* in ways of achieving peak physical performance in the Olympic athlete sense, but to show something of the training methods developed and used in a time before scientific analysis had entered into the *karateka*'s vocabulary.

This book is as much an homage to those who have gone before us and who laid the foundations for the traditional training so many people around the world still find value in, to this day, as it is a manual of physical training. Like every other aspect of *karate*, *hojo undo* requires us to look beyond the physical, to look inward to our own sense of ingenuity and creativity, and to draw upon such attributes to make progress—to cultivate the virtues of hard work and patience. In the mind of those serious about their training, *hojo undo* will always bring to mind the maxim: "*Karate* does not cultivate a person's true character; it reveals it."

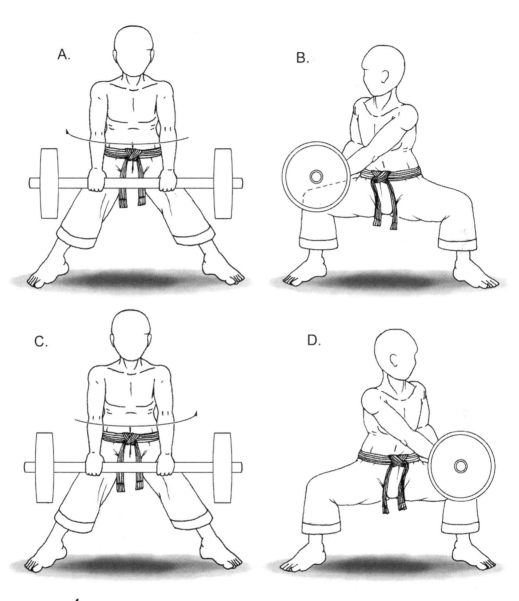

A.

B.

C.

D.

Exercise 1

After lifting the *tan*, with a straight back and using the leg muscles to take the strain, stand with the legs wide enough apart to be able to drop into *shiko dachi*, holding the *tan* as shown in the starting position (Figure A). This exercise focuses on the torso, the leg muscles of the upper thigh, and the connection between these and the postures often found in *kata* from the *Naha-te* tradition, such as *seiyunchin* and *sanseiru*, and from *Shuri-te*, *naihanchin*, or *tekki*, as that series of *kata* are known outside Okinawa.

From the starting position, inhale first before twisting to the right and dropping into *shiko dachi* (Figure B). Exhaling with the drop, the outward breath, the body dropping, and the twist all end at the same time. Take care not to allow the rear leg to buckle. While you turn to the right and sit in *shiko dachi*, the left leg tends to buckle. You must push it back and try to maintain a correct *shiko dachi* posture. Reverse the movement by straightening the legs (Figure C), inhaling through the nose, and twisting the body to the opposite side (Figure D). Again, remember to keep both legs locked into a good stance.

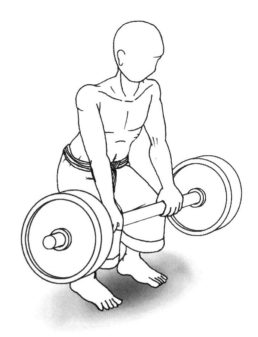

Keep the back straight and remember to let the legs do the lifting.

The inhalation lasts until the body is upright (halfway through the maneuver) before becoming an exhalation through the mouth. Once again, the movement and the breath should end in synchronized harmony. The continuous rising and falling works the legs in the same way as squatting, while the twisting of the torso improves also strength in that part of the body. Take care not to over twist or let the rear leg buckle inward.

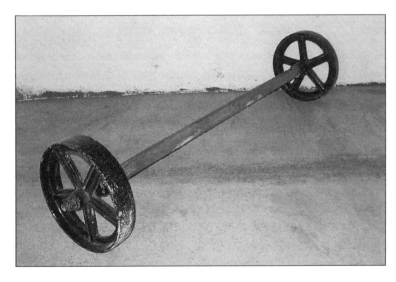

A traditional *tan* made from wood and two iron wheels. This *tan* was made by Richard Barett and is used in his private dojo in Almeria, Spain.

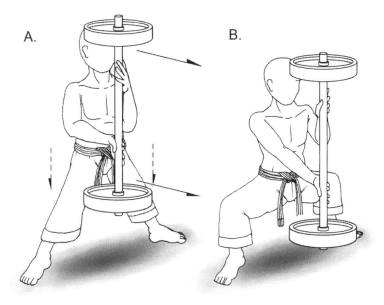

A.

B.

Exercise 2

Holding the *tan* with the hands pointing in opposite directions along the shaft, assume the starting posture with the tool held in a vertical position, close to the body, and the armpits closed (Figure A). Inhale before dropping into *shiko dachi*, straightening the arms while you do so (Figure B). This mimics the *tora uchi* (tiger strike) technique found in many *kata*.

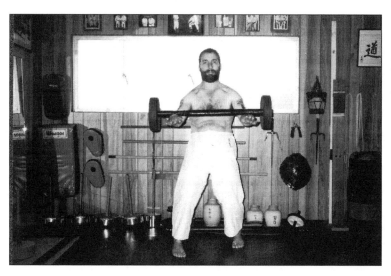

The author, aged 40, conditioning his forearms with the *tan* at his Shinseidokan *dojo* in Perth, Western Australia in 1995.

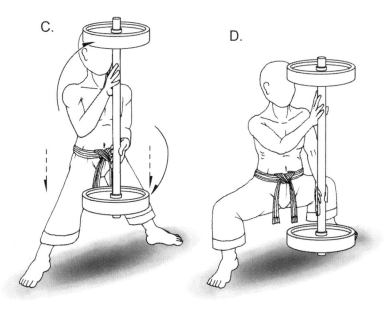

Reverse the movement by standing up while inhaling, drawing the arms back toward the body, mimicking the *mawashi uke* (two-handed swinging block) and twisting the *tan* 180 degrees (Figure C). Then drop back into *shiko dachi* and straighten the arms once more, while exhaling (Figure D). Keep the elbows tucked in and the armpits closed as much as possible throughout the exercise.

A rhythmical and continuous movement should be maintained until the anticipated number of repetitions has been successfully completed, remembering all the time that the challenge is as much a mental one as it is physical. Start with a small number of repetitions and then, as time passes and strength levels improve, increase that number to a maximum of ten in any one set. The link between this exercise and the *mawashi uke/tora uchi* combination found in many *kata* is a clear one, and a strong sense of visualizing this technique can often help when the weight of the *tan* is beginning to make its presence felt through the buildup of lactic acid in tired muscles.

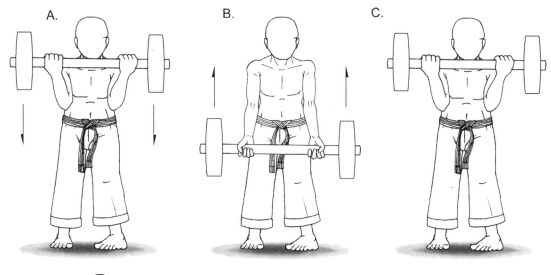

A.   B.   C.

Exercise 3

Adopting a *sanchin dachi*, hold the *tan* in both hands as shown (Figure A). With the elbows tucked in and supported by the front of the body, inhale through the nose, and then lower the forearms while the breath is released and timed to end when the arms reach their full drop (Figure B). Inhale sharply and at the same time return the arms to the starting posture (Figure C). Harmony of breath and body movement is essential, as is the adoption of a correct stance. Having completed the maneuver, step forward into *sanchin dachi* in a slow and deliberate manner before repeating the exercise. *Sanchin kata* footwork (*embusen*) can be followed (but without the turn) or you can simply decide on a number of steps backward and forward, and complete them. Either way, the arms, particularly the bicep and tricep muscles of the upper arm, receive a powerful workout and become all the stronger as a result.

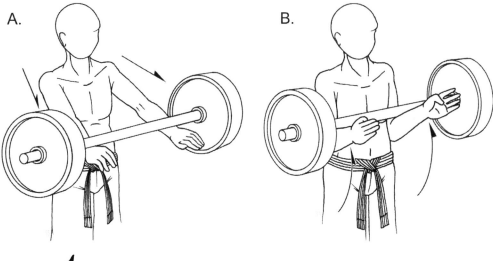

A.

B.

Exercise 4

Standing in *sanchin dachi,* this exercise begins with the *tan* resting on the back of the forearm with the arms held out in front of the body. From this position, the arms are lowered slowly, allowing the *tan* to roll toward the wrists (Figure A). Turning the palms toward each other and the hands slightly upward to check the *tan,* tilt the forearms back, and allow the elbows to drop a little, thus letting the *tan* roll back toward the body (Figure B). Step forward into *sanchin dachi,* and repeat the exercise.

A variation in this exercise can be done by turning the arms on their side, with the palms of the hands facing each other, and following the same maneuver. However, under no circumstances should the *tan* be allowed to roll on the inner forearms. The proximity of the body's blood supply and lack of protective musculature makes this zone a no-go for such punishing training. It is, however, a target we all need to keep in mind when defending against others. A well-placed pinch or grab here from fingers that have been strengthened by training in *hojo undo* is a very powerful weapon indeed.

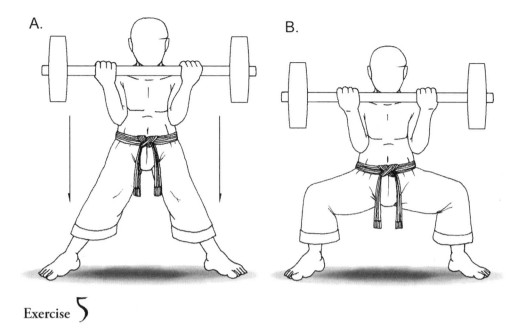

A.

B.

Exercise 5

Begin by holding the *tan* with the legs open wide enough to allow the body to drop into *shiko dachi* (Figure A). Inhale through the nose; while the body drops, strengthen the legs and maintain a straight back (Figure B). Do not allow the spine to curve or the shoulders and hips to become misaligned. The posture adopted should be the same as the one used in *kata*, and no deeper. While focusing the mind on the leg muscles in the thigh, hold the position for a few seconds before exhaling through the open mouth and, at the same time, pushing the legs straight. This movement brings a return to the starting position (Figure A) from where the desired number of repetitions can be made.

Keep in mind that the breath and the accompanying body movement must be made to start and stop at exactly the same time. In other words, the body and the breath should be working together. To do this successfully, you must concentrate at first; however, as the strength and skill levels increase this becomes less an act of concentration and more a sense of understanding. Thus, the trinity of mind, body, and spirit that traditional martial artists strive for is repeatedly manifest in your actions.

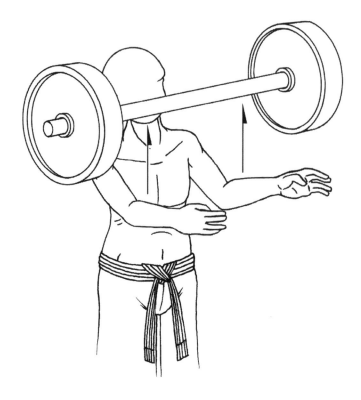

Exercise *6*

Stand in *sanchin dachi* (hourglass posture), palms facing each other with the *tan* resting across the "thumb" edge of the forearms close to the elbow joint. From here, lower the hands and allow the tool to roll slowly toward the wrists. When the tool reaches halfway, bring up the forearms sharply and throw the *tan* into the air before catching it again on the same inside edge of the forearms. This takes some practice; be careful to throw the tool only a few inches at first. Once the *tan* can be thrown and caught again without losing balance and without dropping the tool, the height of the throw can be increased. When this happens, make sure to use the legs like the suspension system on a car (shock absorbers) and do not hold them locked when the *tan* returns to the arms. Once a throw and catch has been completed, take three steps forward, or backward, in *sanchin dachi* and throw again. Great care must be taken not to allow the *tan* to land on the inside of the elbow joint.

Tan Construction Notes

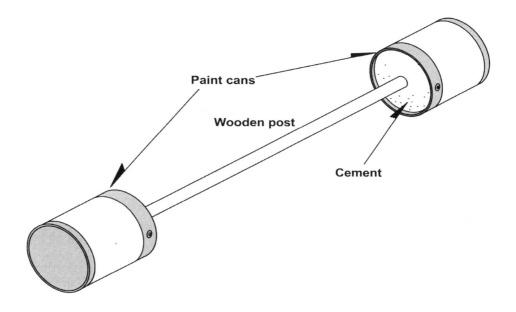

Paint cans

Wooden post

Cement

A construction method similar to the double-handle *chiishi* is used here.

The most common items used in the construction of the *tan* in olden times were a couple of rocks of equal weight, and later, iron wheels, the kind that could be found on the carts and wagons that moved freight around the warehouses and wharfs of Chinese and Okinawan harbors. These days it is often possible to find such wheels on farms and at country markets, or in junk shops. In fact, the latter is where I found a number of the tools used in my *dojo*. Again, if iron wheels cannot be found, use standard weights from a sports shop. Place the weight at each end of a round pole of solid strong wood, similar to oak, approximately four feet (122 cm) in length. Make sure that the weight is securely fixed to each end and the wooden shaft is strong enough to take the weight. If buying weights is not an option, then using two old paint cans as molds can make a perfectly good *tan*. Fill them with cement, attaching them to both ends of a stout post in a similar way to the *chiishi* construction method and remove once the cement is set. The *tan* in my *dojo* weighs 34 lbs. (15 kg).

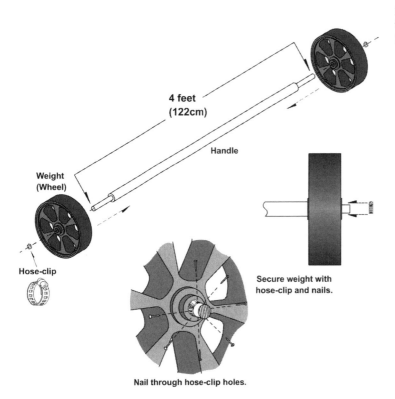

Iron wheels from farms or industrial sources make a perfect *tan*.

4 feet (122cm)

Handle

Weight (Wheel)

Hose-clip

Secure weight with hose-clip and nails.

Nail through hose-clip holes.

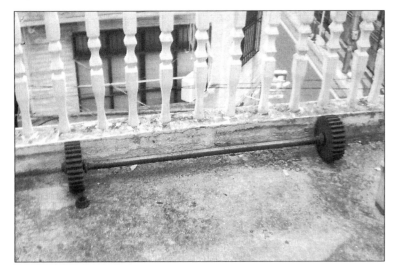

During a visit to the Meibu-kan *dojo* in Kume, Okinawa, the author spotted this *tan* made from heavy-duty engine gears.

Ishisashi – Stone Lock

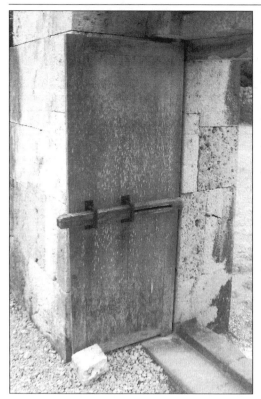

The original use of the *sashi* can be seen in this photograph. Although these 'modern' *sashi* are made from iron, in former times they would have been made from carved stones.

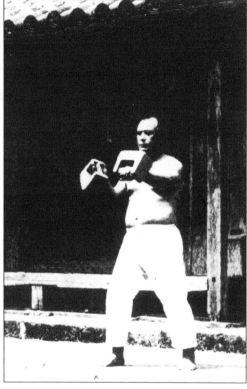

The author's teacher, Eiichi Miyazato *sensei*, training in *sanchin kata* with the *ishisashi*.

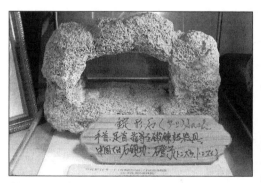

This ancient *ishi sashi*, carved from solid rock, is on display at the Okinawa Karate Museum in Nishihara.

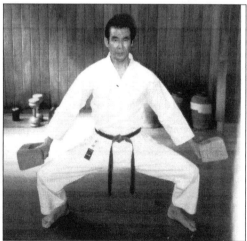

Tetsunosuke Yasuda *sensei* was in his 70's when this photograph was taken. Now in his mid-eighties, he still trains in *karate*, *iaido* (the art of drawing the sword and making a cut), and yoga, and acts as the senior advisor to the Jundokan *dojo*.

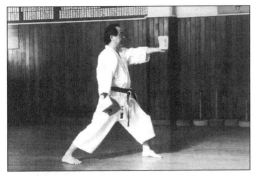

Here Hisao Sunagawa uses the *ishisashi* to enhance his shoulder strength by recreating the postures and movements found in the *Goju ryu kata, shisochin*.

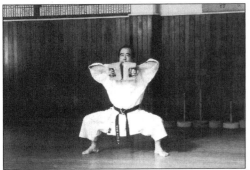

Hisao Sunagawa of the Jundokan *dojo*, Okinawa, uses the *ishisashi* to help develop his excellent *shiko dachi* (low stance), as well as his shoulder muscles.

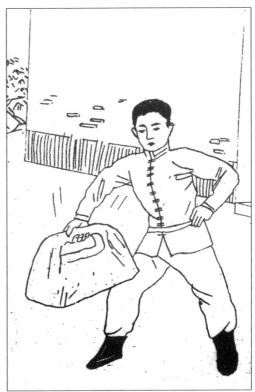

A single giant *ishisashi* appears in this old Chinese martial arts manual, a copy of which was given to the author some years ago by Tetsuhiro Hokama *sensei*, the owner and proprietor of the Okinawa Karate Museum.

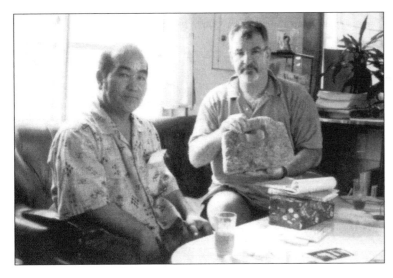

Karate teacher, historian and world renowned author, Patrick McCarthy discussing *hojo undo* with Masahiro Nakamoto at his home in Shuri, Okinawa.

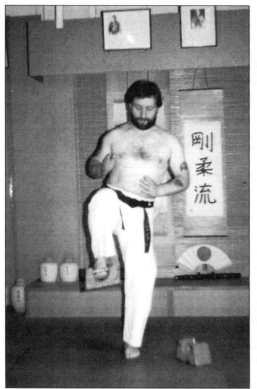

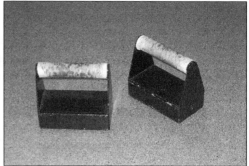

These *tetsu sashi* belong to the author.

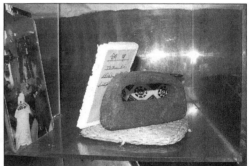

The author strengthening his legs with a heavy set of *tetsu sashi* at his Jinseido *dojo* in Devon, England c. 1985.

Tetsu sashi, *sashi* made from iron on display at the Okinawa Karate Museum, Nishihara.

As the name suggests, the *ishi* (stone) *sashi* (lock) is yet another example of the way nature and everyday items the *karateka* found around them provided objects of resistance for Okinawan *karateka* to work with. Stone has always been in abundance on the rocky island outcrop and has played an important role in the local construction of buildings from the earliest days of settlement. The *ishisashi* was designed to fit on a door or gateway and acted as a locking mechanism by allowing a length of wood to be passed through the handles. A double door with a *sashi* on each one and a heavy post passing through the two of them made a very effective lock. In modern times, *sashi* made from stone became rarer and were replaced by door fittings made from iron. As stone locks fell from use they found a second life in the *dojo*[11] being set up all over Okinawa. Today, however, finding stone *sashi* in a *dojo* is exceptional, as here, too, tools made from iron have replaced them. At the *Jundokan dojo* where I train when I am in Okinawa, many of the tools used came directly from Chojun Miyagi's *dojo*. The Miyagi family presented them to Eiichi Miyazato when the *Jundokan* was established in 1957. Three *sashi* carved from solid stone are still in use there today, and I never fail to work out with them during my visits. Even so, the material used to make these tools is not important. What is important is that each tool is made well and used properly. By following these two rules, *karateka* are free to focus their attention on the training itself.

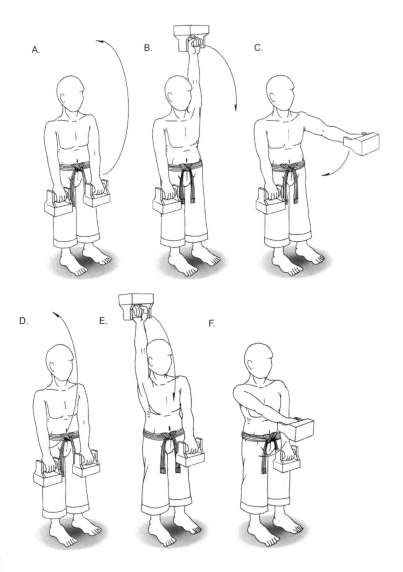

A.

B.

C.

D.

E.

F.

Exercise 1

Standing in *heiko dachi*, hold the *sashi* in front of the body with the palms facing in toward the body as shown (Figure A). Keeping the arms straight at all times, raise the left arm in an arc until it points vertically above the head (Figure B). The movement should be matched exactly with an inhalation through the nose that starts and finishes with the lift. From there the tool is lowered halfway while half the breath is released (Figure C). A pause and brief moment of focusing both the arm and the breath is taken before continuing with the return of the tool to its original position, accompanied by the complete exhalation of the breath. From there, the action is repeated with the right arm.

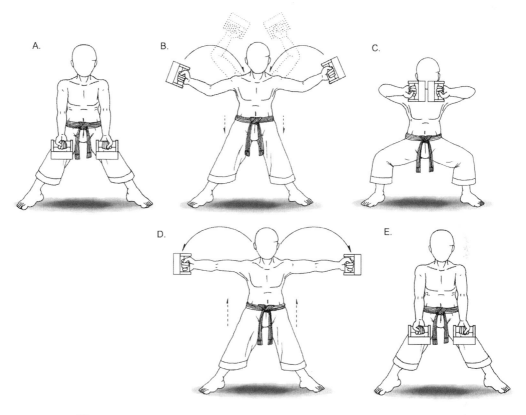

Exercise 2

Standing with the legs open wide enough to sit into *shiko dachi* and with the palms of the hands facing outward away from the body (Figure A), swing both arms out to the side in a large arcing movement (Figure B) until the tools come together. At that point, and without a pause, the body drops into *shiko dachi* with the *sashi* coming to rest in the position shown in front of the body (Figure C). All this is accomplished on a single inhalation that should blend seamlessly with the movement. Hold for no more than a second or two before reversing the arm movement; standing back up and beginning the exhalation, stop the *sashi* at the halfway point (Figure D). The breath is also checked before the movement continues and the last of the outward breath is released when you return to the starting position (Figure E).

In both of the first two exercises, particular attention should be paid to the *latissimus dorsi* muscles (the "lats") when stopping the tool halfway through the exhalation. Bringing the tool to a halt by closing down the armpit and contracting this muscle is the desired objective and helps develop a strong feeling of connection to the techniques of *sanchin* and other *kata*. Being able to remember these exercises alone is not the same as gaining a lasting benefit from them. For that, you must develop a "feeling" for each tool, and in much the same way as a weapon becomes an extension of a trained person's body, the tools of *hojo undo* should eventually fade from focus in the mind of the person using them. Only then can their manipulation become natural and without stress, and the degree to which a person's ability to withstand such stress becomes evident.

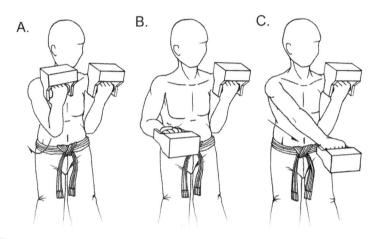

Exercise *3*

Adopting *sanchin dachi*, left leg forward and making a double *chudan uke* posture (Figure A), the *sashi* is held tight and not allowed to slip through the fingers. Keeping the body of the tool in line with the forearm at all times works the fingers and the gripping action of the hand and may, at first, prove a little difficult. Perseverance is the key here; remember that it is the mind as well as the body being challenged.

Withdraw the right arm slowly as if pulling something heavy (Figure B) and inhale through the nose. Reverse the breath, this time through the mouth, and punch the arm out slowly and deliberately (Figure C), not forgetting to add the twisting action found in a normal *karate* punch. The punch and exhalation end together before the arm is returned to the *chudan uke* position. This return action, although a short one, should be accompanied by a faster inhalation and exhalation. Ending in the original start position (Figure A) at the end of an exhalation, step forward with the left leg and repeat the exercise with the right arm.

This stepping and punching can be continued in a straight line, or, as with the *nigiri gami*, the *embusen* of *sanchin kata* can be followed.

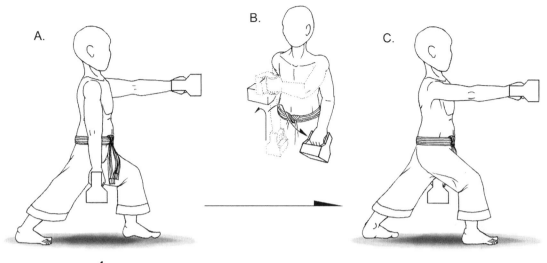

A.

B.

C.

Exercise 4

Holding a *sashi* in each hand, step forward into *zenkutsu dachi*, punching one hand out to the front while pulling the other arm down to the side (Figure A). Stepping forward, also into *zenkutsu dachi*, the punching arm swings across the front of the body in an arc before coming to a stop at the side of the leg, while the other arm lifts up the *sashi* along the side of the body and thrusts to the front (Figure B) in a slow punching action. Both arm movements begin and end at the same time, inhaling for the first part of the movement before exhaling while the blocking arm swings across the front of the body and downward, and the punching arm thrusts forward (Figure C). At that point, the legs and body are momentarily tensed when the breath is fully exhaled.

Relax the body and step forward into *zenkutsu dachi* with the other leg while repeating the arm actions. Take only two or three steps in this fashion before changing direction either to the side or the rear by use of *mawate* (about face) turning. Walking backward is also practiced in this exercise, but regardless of the direction taken, the movements should be smooth and the breathing switching from inhalation to exhalation as seamlessly as possible. Keep the shoulders down, the armpits closed, and focus on the *tanden* to facilitate the breath.

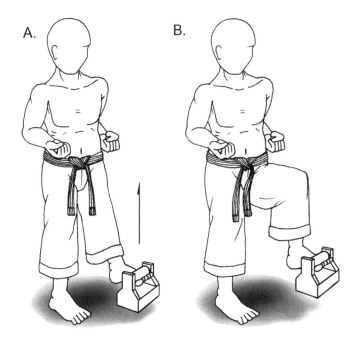

A.   B.

Exercise 5

Slipping a foot into one of the *sashi*, raise the knee and slowly lower it down again. This exercise is not only a workout for the muscles of the leg, but is a good test of your balance too. You will soon discover that a correct alignment of your body's weight is an essential precursor to this exercise. Simply by lifting the leg carrying the *sashi* up and down tests the balance of those new to such training while allowing a certain amount of acclimatization to the tool before moving on to more challenging exercises.

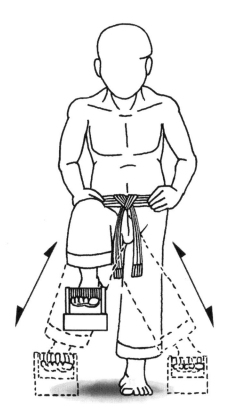

Exercise 6

A similar but more challenging exercise with the *sashi* is to lift the tool with the foot as in Exercise Five; only this time cross the leg over the front of the body as if kicking with a low side kick (*yoko geri*) before raising the knee back up and then kicking out to the side in a similar fashion. The kick across the front of the body stimulates your sense of balance, while the kick to the side is the same as that required at the start of the *Goju ryu kata kururunfa*, and also found within *sanseiru*, and *seisan*,[12] when a low side kick is executed and followed up immediately by crossing the kicking leg in front of the body to place the foot back on the ground before twisting into a tight 180-degree turn.

Ishisashi Construction Notes

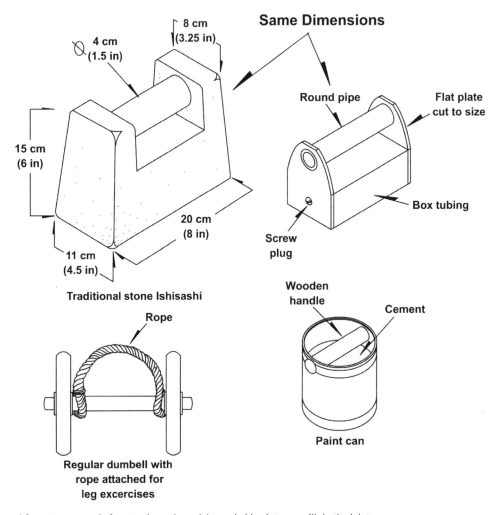

Same Dimensions

4 cm (1.5 in)

8 cm (3.25 in)

15 cm (6 in)

11 cm (4.5 in)

20 cm (8 in)

Traditional stone Ishisashi

Round pipe

Flat plate cut to size

Box tubing

Screw plug

Wooden handle

Cement

Paint can

Rope

Regular dumbell with rope attached for leg excercises

Carved from stone or made from steel, regular weights and old paint cans will do the job too.

These tools take a little imagination to construct and access to a stonemason or someone with a workshop and abilities in welding. However, I have seen versions of *ishisashi* made from old paint cans filled with cement and given wooden handles, as well as house bricks with wire handles fixed to them. If it is not possible to fashion the traditional tools from stone or from metal, it is possible to train in all these exercises with a suitably weighted set of dumbbells. A short length of rope tied to the dumbbell facilitates the leg exercise. The *sashi* I use are made from lengths of steel box pipe, tube, and plate, welded together; they weigh 8 lbs. each (4.5 kg). A small hole at one end (plugged by a screw) allows sand to be added, increasing the weight of the tool.

Kongoken – Large Iron Ring

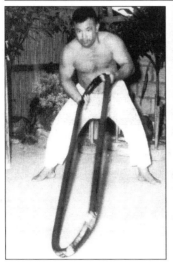 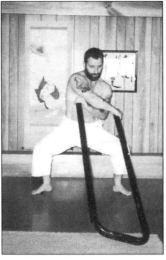 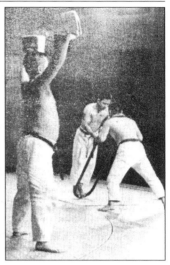

The author's teacher, Eiichi Miyazato *sensei*. This photograph was taken around 1960 when he was approaching 40 years of age. His *judo*, as well as his *karate*, no doubt benefited from training with the *kongoken*.

The author at 40 years of age, wrestling with the *kongoken* at his *dojo* in Perth, Western Australia.

With the *ishisashi* being demonstrated by a student of the Jundokan in the foreground of this photograph, a two-person *kongoken* drill is under way in the background. Naha, October 1973.

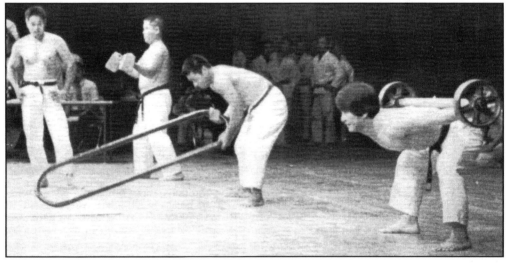

Here, Ryosei Arakaki looks on while his fellow Jundokan students display the *ishisashi*, *kongoken*, and *tan*. Naha, October 1973.

In the mid 1930s, Chojun Miyagi *sensei*, the founder of *Goju ryu karatedo*, traveled to the Hawaiian Islands in the mid-Pacific to teach *karate* and to lecture on its history and cultural benefits.[13] During his time there, he observed the local wrestlers training.

Stopping to observe their methods, he noticed the use of a large and obviously heavy iron ring. Almost as tall as a man and weighing anything from 45 lbs. (20 kg) up to 80 lbs. (35 kg), it was being used by one and sometimes two wrestlers in ways that captured the

karate master's imagination. So impressed was he by the training aid, legend has it he brought one or more home with him on his return to Okinawa in the early part of 1935.[14] The original use of the *kongoken* is now lost and open to speculation. However, through my correspondence with Charles C. Goodin[15] in Hawaii, I concur with his suggestion that it is most likely these heavy loops of iron were used initially as either ship's ballast or in some way connected to the crushing of sugar cane, a crop that has been cultivated extensively on the islands since they were first occupied around A.D. 600. Later European occupation brought with it mechanization and modern extraction methods and as a result the farming of sugar became an important export industry for the islands.

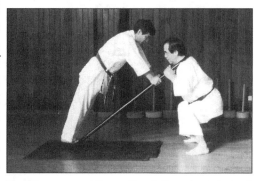

Hisao Sunagawa and Kazuya Higa, both senior students of the Jundokan *dojo* in Okinawa, working with the *kongoken* to increase leg strength. Both men, friends and contemporaries of the author, are in their 50's.

Those who worked the cane fields, however, came mainly from the lower economic strata of Hawaiian society, and it is unlikely that such people would have had access to whatever first-class training equipment existed at the time. If interested in any form of pugilism, individuals would have undoubtedly made use of the things they came into contact with during the course of their everyday working lives. Regardless of what the *kongoken* was originally used for, in the hands of Hawaiian wrestlers or the *karateka* back on Okinawa, it became yet one more tool in an arsenal of training devices employed to help them develop the kind of strength and power they were looking for to complement their fighting technique.

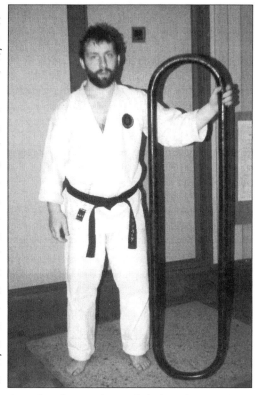

The author after a workout with the kongoken at Morio Higaonna sensei's dojo in Kiyose, Tokyo in 1986.

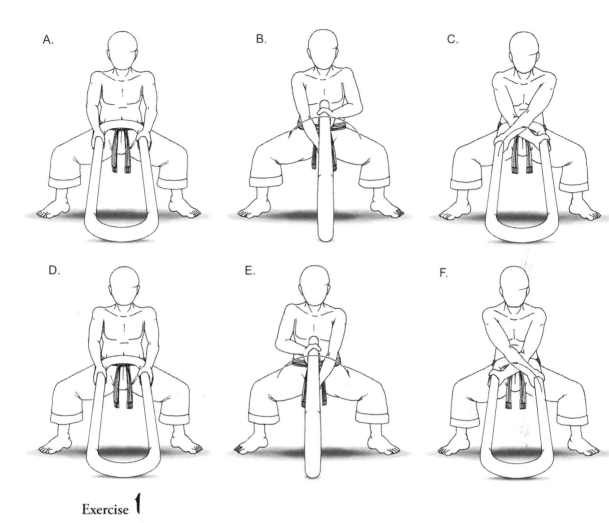

A. B. C.

D. E. F.

Exercise 1

Begin by holding the *kongoken* as shown (Figure A). Making sure your back is up-right and the legs strong, allow the tool to slip through the fingers and palm of the hand while the left arm pushes over and the right arm pushes under (Figure B), thus twisting the tool on its own axis. With the arms now crossed (Figure C), both of them pull in a reverse motion returning to the starting position (Figure D) and continue through twisting the tool to the opposite side (Figures E and F) before once more reversing. It is important not to stop there, however, but to continue by pushing and pulling in a continuous motion, back and forth, from one side to the other. The movement of the arms being crossed on one side to being crossed over and back again counts as one exercise. If possible, you should try to begin by completing at least fifty. Do not allow the legs to come up out of a strong *shiko dachi*. Regardless of how difficult this exercise might seem in the beginning, you should remember that with one end of the tool remaining on the ground, only a portion of its true weight is being dealt with.

As always, the breath is a vital partner in how the tool is manipulated and should be utilized as seamlessly as possible. In short, an inhalation accompanies every pulling action of the arms and an exhalation accompanies every pushing action. Try to synchronize your breathing with your movements. If you move too quickly, it becomes difficult to breathe and results in the exercise coming to a halt. Successfully harmonizing the physical action with the breath makes the tool seem to move almost by itself. Use brute force and the tool always wins. Moreover, a final word of caution—if you are doing this exercise on a wooden floor, be sure you use a rubber mat or some kind of carpet to protect the floor.

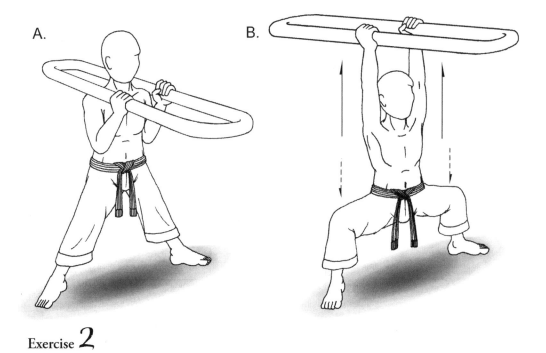

A.

B.

Exercise 2

In this exercise, the aim is to use explosive power to lift the *kongoken* above the head. Begin by finding the balance point along the center of the *kongoken*, bend the knees, and allow the tool to come to rest above the shoulders. Standing with the feet wide enough to allow a drop into *shiko dachi* and with the *kongoken* balanced in the hands (Figure A), take in a deep breath. With as forceful exhalations as possible emanating from the *tanden*, drop into *shiko dachi* and thrust the tool above the head (Figure B). Hold this position for two or three seconds before relaxing back into the upright position and allowing the *kongoken* to come back down to shoulder height. Should either be necessary, re-adjust your stance or the balance of the *kongoken* before executing another lift. If possible, this exercise should consist of three sets of six lifts, with each set separated by a one-minute rest.

A.

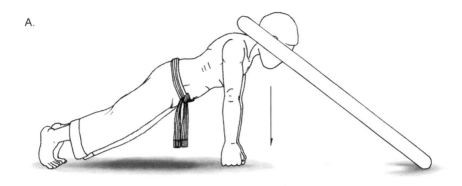

B.

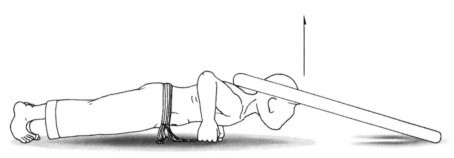

Exercise 3

Assume a normal push-up position—experienced *karateka* should be on their first two knuckles. See Figure A on page 156 about push-ups in the chapter about auxilliary exercises. Have a partner place one end of the *kongoken* over the head, resting on the neck. From this position, execute ten push-ups before the tool is removed for a thirty-second break. At least three sets of ten push-ups should be done each time to feel any benefit. The stronger you become, the more sets you can schedule into the exercise.

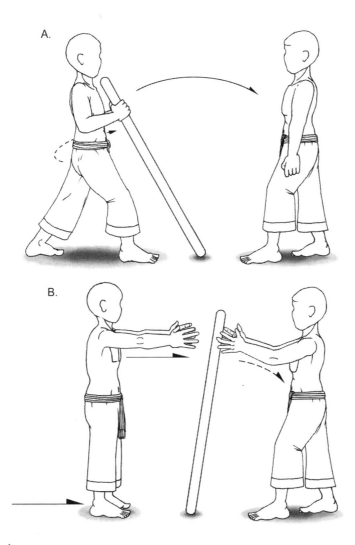

A.

B.

Exercise 4

The next two exercises are aimed at working the tool with a partner. Both people should be familiar with the tool and be able to handle its weight. Standing in *heiko dachi* (natural stance) an equal distance from the *kongoken* (Figure A), the idea is to use explosive power to throw the tool away and into the hands of your partner. Try not to grab at the tool too tightly; rather, leave the hands open and relaxed but prepared, and use the arms as shock absorbers to help dissipate the incoming force when the *kongoken* comes your way. Be careful to guard the face from impact by timing the "catch" with the speed of the approaching tool and taking a small step backward. When the *kongoken* begins to approach, reach out to meet it and let the sides of the tool fall into the open palms of both hands. Bend the arms and step backward. This

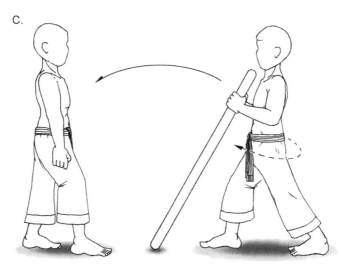

C.

receiving action is done with an accompanying inhalation that ends at the same time as the physical movement. When throwing the tool, care should be taken to coordinate the rear leg, the arms, and the strong exhalation that accompanies each throw. Remember to breathe out by contracting the *tanden* and not the upper chest. The rear leg is brought sharply back up to *heiko dachi* by the use of a powerful push from the hip, while at the same time the arms thrust out like two hydraulic rams (Figure B). Both actions are done while breathing out and focusing the *tanden*.

When the *kongoken* returns, step back with the opposite leg each time and repeat the catching and throwing exercise with the opposite side of the body (Figure C). The aim is to build explosive power over a very short distance with only a small movement, using the thrust of the hips (*koshi*). At first, try to complete fifty throws, eventually leading to one hundred or more when the skill and feeling for what you are doing improves.

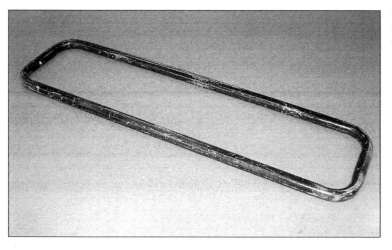

The author's *kongoken* at the Shinseidokan *dojo*. It weighs 50 lbs. (23 kg).

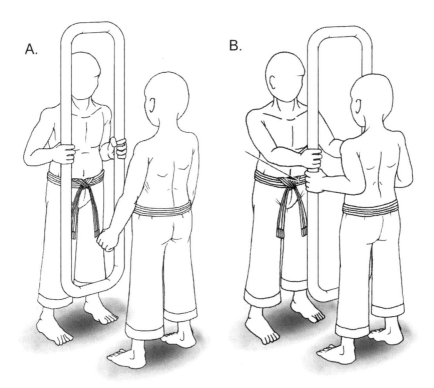

A.

B.

Exercise 5

Stand in *heiko dachi* facing a partner holding the *kongoken* close to the chest as shown (Figure A). One person always grabs on the top, and the other always grabs on the bottom; you should decide which before the exercise starts. Thrust the *kongoken* out toward your partner, who in turn should reach out and take it (Figure B).

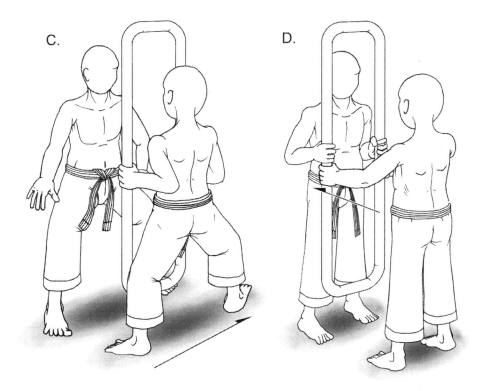

Both then use *tai sabaki* (body shifting) to slide to the side (Figure C) before the tool is handed back (Figure D). A second body shift, back to the original positions, is done before the *kongoken* is once more handed back to your partner. This sliding back and forth and the handing over of the tool should be done at least ten times in one set. A short rest in between sets is needed. The number of sets depends on the strength, skill, and determination of the two people involved. Correct breathing, as always, is essential if the tool is not to take over and bring you to a premature standstill. Inhale when you accept the tool, slide quickly to one side, and then exhale (completely) when you hand the tool back. This exercise tests your breath control after only a few exchanges. If it is not in harmony with the movement, it stops you in your tracks.

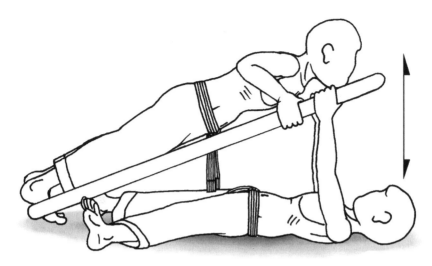

Exercise *6*

One person lies on his back with his legs spread open, holding the *kongoken* as if doing a bench press. His training partner then places his feet on the end of the tool and puts his hands onto the *kongoken*. The further toward the top of the *kongoken* the partner places his hands, the heavier and more challenging this exercise is for the person on the ground. From this position, the person doing the lift takes a deep breath in through the nose and, with exhalation, pushes the *kongoken* and his training partner up until the arms are outstretched. Once this is done, bend the arms and lower the tool and your partner back down with care and control. Once you become used to this exercise, it can be done in a slow and confident rhythm until a desired number of repetitions have been completed.

When working at first with this tool, it is advisable to have a training partner who is able to assist should the weight become unmanageable. Having two people working together also allows one person to rest while the other is working the tool. Each person can be an effective source of encouragement to the other when the going gets tough and the number of repetitions begins to undergo a mental review when fatigue starts setting in.

Kongoken Construction Notes

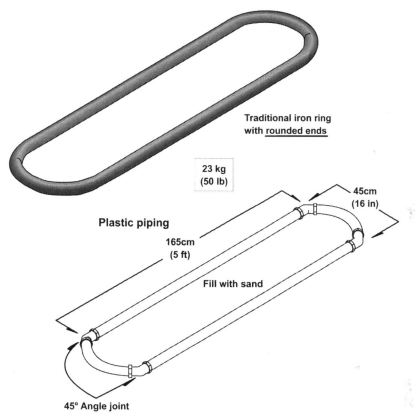

Traditional iron ring
with <u>rounded ends</u>

23 kg
(50 lb)

45cm
(16 in)

Plastic piping

165cm
(5 ft)

Fill with sand

45° Angle joint

Seriously heavy or made from plastic pipe and sand, construct a tool that will challenge all who pick it up.

Again, it might prove difficult to obtain this tool, difficult, but not impossible! My first *kongoken* was made from household plastic plumber's pipe filled with sand. However, serious training requires a serious tool and a heavy ring of iron or steel tubing must be found at some point. Fabrication and engineering factories are a good place to go. If you approach them with the right attitude and ask for assistance, it is possible to acquire a *kongoken* that outlives the owner. Between five and five and one-half feet (150-165 cm) in length, it should be wide enough to allow your head to fit comfortably in between each of the sides when you rest the tool on your shoulders. Traditionally, the tool should approximate the weight of another person. In my *dojo*, the *kongoken* weighs 50 lbs. (23 kg).

Tetsu Geta – Iron Sandal

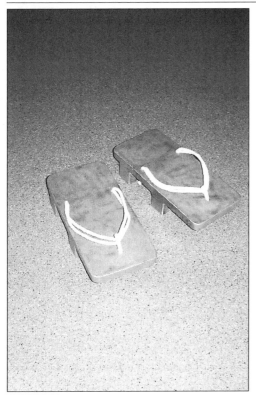

The author's *tetsu geta* weigh around 12 lbs., or 5 kg.

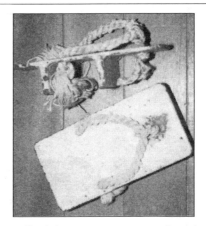

Iron *geta*, like their stone counterparts, can be made as heavy or as light as required. This old pair on display at the Okinawa Karate Museum shows they do not always have to be very heavy.

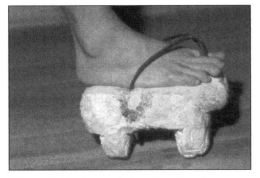

This remarkable photograph shows the extraordinary lengths to which the Okinawans went to enhance their *karate* by utilizing the resources they had around them as in this case the local stone and some old fence wire. Nothing was ever 'store bought'.

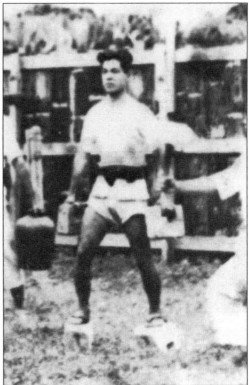

Perhaps he was just posing for the camera or perhaps not? Either way the *karateka* in this photograph, taken at the Kenkyukai *dojo* in Naha, c. 1928, has a lot to deal with while he uses both the *ishisashi* and *ishi geta* at the same time.

These days, you rarely find this training tool made out of its original material: stone (*ishi geta*). Instead, those who still use it, train with sandals made from iron (*tetsu geta*). The varieties of exercises you can do with this tool are limited, and most of them can be done just as well with the *ishisashi* or with the use of modern ankle weights. Where the traditional *geta* made from either stone or iron still holds its own, however, is in the nature of the focus it brings to bear on the toes. When kicking your height, for example, the toes must grip the cord tightly to avoid the effects of the centrifugal forces involved from throwing the heavy *geta* from the foot. Using the *geta* also helps develop your balance, and this, along with the increased strength in the leg muscles, gives value to the continued use of this tool. All the kicks found in traditional *karate* can be practiced, with various levels of modification, while wearing the stone or iron *geta*. However, I would recommend that great care be taken until you get used to the challenges this tool presents to your balance. Slow and steady progress is the key.

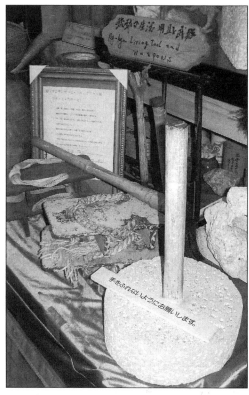

A beautiful old *chiishi* stands next to two different pairs of *tetsu geta* at the Okinawa Karate Museum.

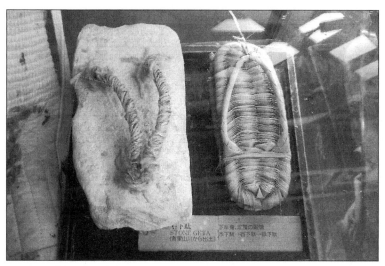

Compare the *karate ishi geta* on the left, made from stone, with the normal *geta* on the right made from woven straw. Both are on display at the Okinawa Karate Museum in Nishihara.

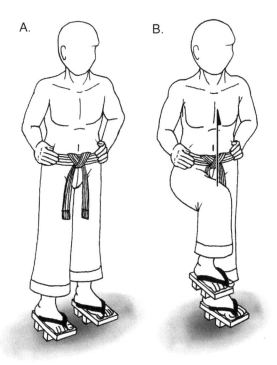

A.   B.

Exercise 1

Wearing both *geta* and with the hands on the hips (Figure A), lift the knee as quickly as possible, as if kicking using the *heiza geri* (knee kick) technique (Figure B). Repeat this in three sets of ten before changing to the other leg. This exercise is not done in the same relaxed manner as Exercise Five with the *ishisashi*. Instead, grip the *geta* with the toes and use the legs as if you were kicking with the foot exploding from the ground as fast as you can move it.

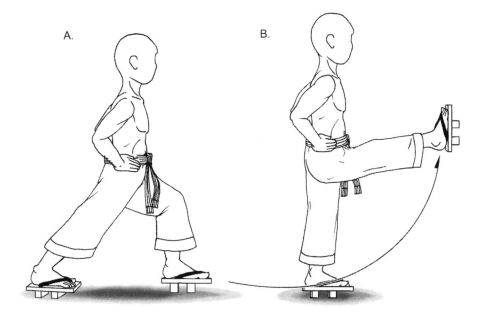

A.

B.

Exercise 2

Standing in *zenkutsu dachi* (forward stance), again with the hands placed on the hips (Figure A), proceed to swing the rear leg up and to the front while keeping it straight (Figure B) as if kicking your height. Again, repeat this in three sets of ten before changing sides.

It is, of course, also possible to repeat with the *geta* the same leg exercises done with the *ishisashi*. However, with the extra grip afforded by the straps on the *geta*, their main worth is found in the practice of quick, explosive moves and the increased need for good balance that comes with wearing the *geta*.

Tetsu Geta Construction Notes

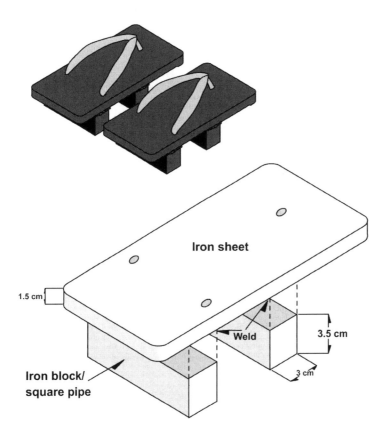

Iron sheet

1.5 cm

Weld

3.5 cm

3 cm

Iron block/
square pipe

Traditional *geta* also develop the gripping power of the toes.

Have two rectangular pieces of steel plate cut to size (this depends on the size of the user's own feet) and drill three holes as indicated on the drawing. Take care to position the top hole in line with the gap between the big toe and the next. Two lengths of square steel rod, equal in length to the width of the rectangular plate being used as the *geta*, are then welded to the plate. Once the metal has cooled completely, the cord should be threaded through the holes from the top and then tied off in a strong knot. Where the cord from each side comes together between the toes, bind the cords as one with more cord or electrical tape. The *geta* can be made with a weight that suits the user, but for the average male adult they should, like the pair in my *dojo*, weigh around 12 lbs. (5 kg).

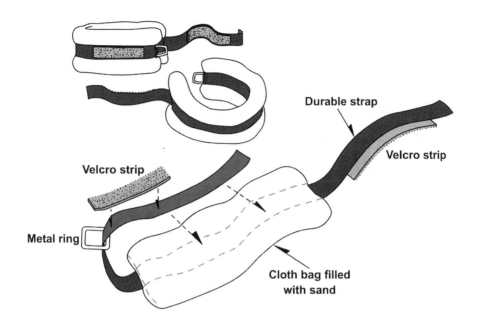

Durable strap

Velcro strip

Velcro strip

Metal ring

Cloth bag filled with sand

Better than nothing at all, ankle weights will build leg strength.

Should it prove impossible to make a pair of iron *geta*, a heavy set of ankle weights approximates the challenges posed by this tool. Unfortunately, ankle weights do little to help strengthen the gripping ability of the toes. Nevertheless, it is important to remember a basic tenet of *hojo undo*: we use what we have at hand to help improve our *karate*. If ankle weights are all you have available to you, then use them.

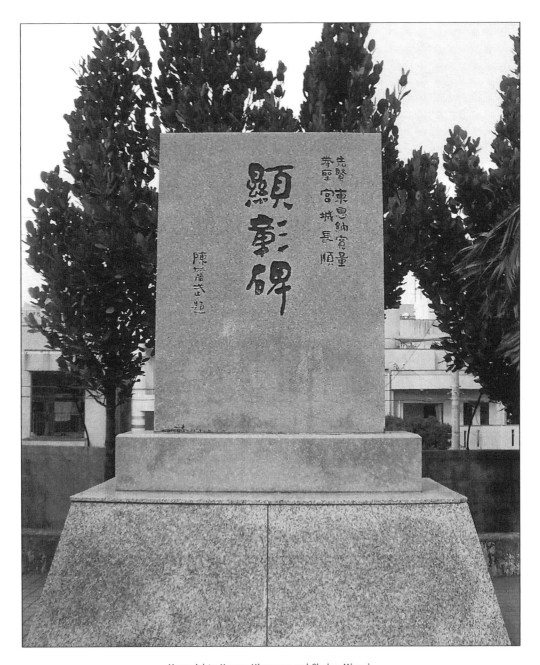

先賢 東恩納寛量
孝聖 宮城長順

顯彰碑

陳信武題

Memorial to Kanryo Higaonna and Chojun Miyagi.

4 IMPACT TOOLS

Unlike the tools discussed up to now, the equipment in this chapter introduces and delivers various levels of shock to the body of the user. Shock, either corporal or psychological, is often the reason why people are brought to a standstill when it comes to getting through a tough situation. When the shock of impact hits and the stress levels begin to climb, this is when *karateka* remind themselves to look for ways through and not waste time searching for ways out. Dealing calmly with shock is an ability acquired by becoming familiar with it, and in this notion lays the reasoning behind the training. No one is suggesting we should grow to enjoy pain or discomfort; on the contrary, as healthy human beings, we should try to minimize such negativity in our lives. However, *karate* is a form of self-defense we will call on in times of high stress and anxiety. It is not the time to "freeze" when our assailant's blows hurt when we block them. Familiarity is the key to being able to cope under stress and working regularly with the following tools will help you find that.

Makiwara – Striking Post

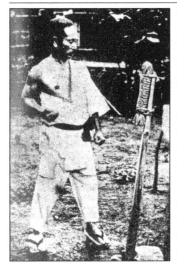 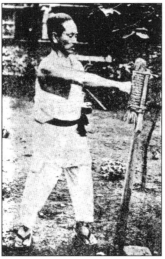 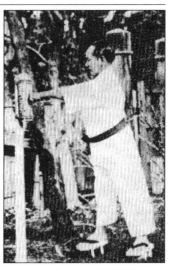

Gichin Funakoshi (1868-1957), with his *do-gi* jacket removed on one side, perhaps to suggest the same solemnity as an archer in *kyudo* (Japanese archery) adopts when facing his target (also known as a *makiwara*). He prepares himself for the punch.

The punch is thrown. Unlike *kyudo* however, in *karate* it is most definitely essential to hit the target.

A very rare photograph of Gichin Funakoshi training with the *makiwara*.

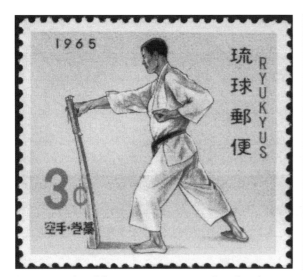 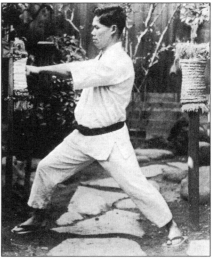

In 1965, a series of three postage stamps were issued, each one depicting an important part of *karate* training. This one clearly shows the importance of *hojo undo* and the *makiwara* in particular.

Surrounded by three *makiwara*, Giko (Yoshitaka) Funakoshi (1906-1945), the third son of Gichin Funakoshi who was according to many historians the person most responsible for modern *Shotokan karate*, uses just one of the tools to train his punch. Unfortunately he died tragically young at the age of 39.

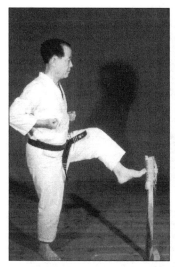

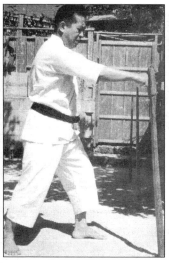

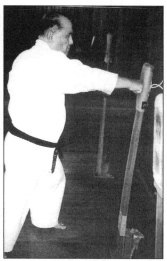

Founder of the Matsubayashi school of *Shorin ryu karate*, the late Shoshin Nagamine (1907-1997) can be seen in this rare photograph training his toes on a *makiwara* especially made for kicking.

Yuchoku Higa (1910-1994) was a strong believer in *hojo undo*. Even when he was in his 70's he would get up at 5.00 A.M. each morning and jog for 5 km before returning to the *dojo* to skip.

Eiichi Miyazato (1922-1999), the late headmaster of the Jundokan *dojo*, still hitting the *makiwara* at the age of 72.

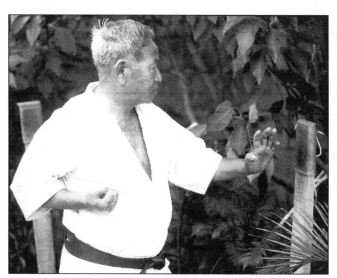

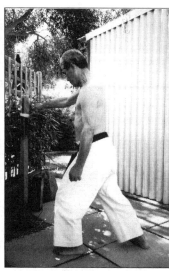

Meitoku Yagi (1912–2003), was a senior student of Chojun Miyagi, the founder of *Goju ryu karate*. After his teacher's death, he opened his own *dojo*, the Meibukan. With many students in Okinawa, Japan, and around the world, he was a very important figure in Okinawan *karate* history.

Kosuke Yonamine (b. 1939) 9th *Dan Uechi ryu karate* and 8th *Dan* Okinawan *kobudo*. Note the lack of *hekite* (pulling back of the non-punching arm) in Yonamine *sensei*'s punching technique. This photograph was taken during his visit to the author's *dojo* in 1997.

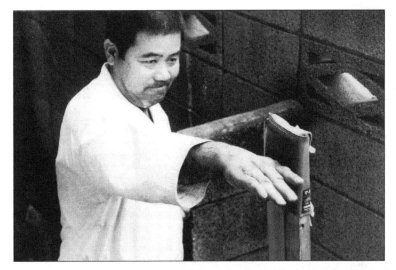

Morio Higaonna (b. 1938) has trained on the *maki-wara* almost all his life. Here he is conditioning the inside ridge of his hand by striking the *makiwara* continually with *heito uchi*.

Tettsui uchi (hammer-fist strike) being used with full force by Morio Higaonna against the *makiwara*.

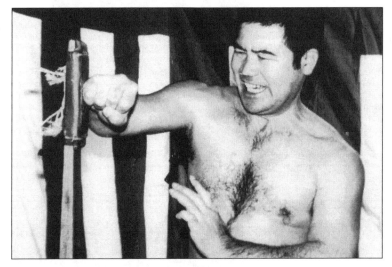

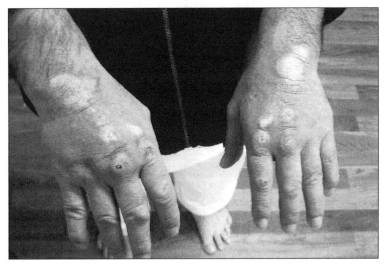

At 70 years of age and with a lifetime of conditioning behind them, these were Morio Higaonna's hands as they looked when the author visited him at his *dojo* in Makishi, Okinawa in February 2008.

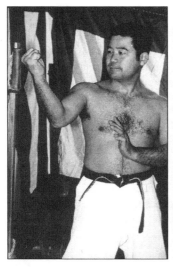

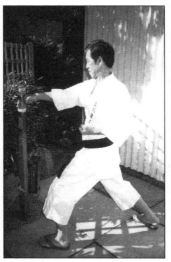

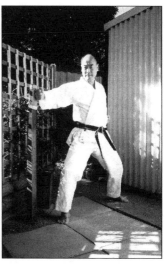

Uraken (back fist) too is slammed into the target when Higaonna *sensei* engages the *makiwara*.

Hirokazu Kanazawa (b. 1931). Perhaps the most famous master of *Shotokan karate* alive in the world today, he is seen here training on the author's *makiwara* at the Shinseidokan *dojo* in 1986.

A front cover for *Shotokan Karate Magazine* (August 1996), Keigo Abe 8th *Dan*. (b. 1938) a legend of the Japan Karate Association and now headmaster of his own school in Japan, here using the author's *makiwara* to practice his *uraken* (back fist strike).

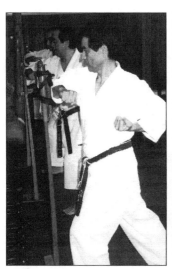

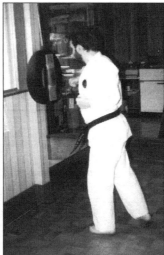

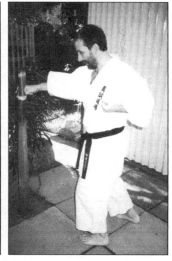

Students at the Jundokan *dojo*, Kazuya Higa, Hisao Sunagawa, and an unknown person use the *makiwara* to work on their *empi* technique, c. 2006.

While training at the Higaonna *dojo* in Kiyose, Tokyo, in 1987, the author learned how to use this type of *makiwara* to practice block and punch combinations—something not really possible with the standard tool.

Punches...nothing fancy, just lots of them. Here the author works his way through the designated number of sets before training begins. Five hundred does not take long to say, but it is a different matter sometimes when the skin splits open.

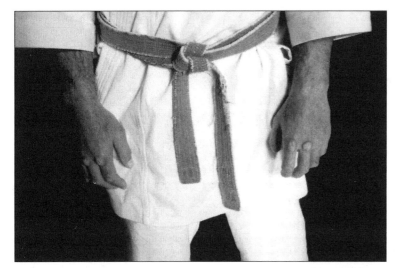

A close up of Masaji Taira's hands indicate the level of training done on the *makiwara*. It should be remembered that large knuckles are not the aim of *makiwara* practice, but a result of it.

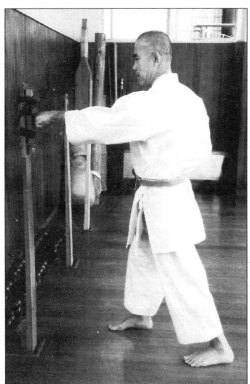

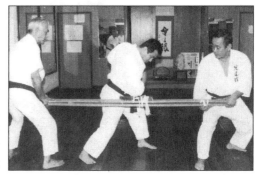

Students of the late Yuchoku Higa training at the Kyudokan *dojo* with a portable *makiwara* constructed in the traditional Okinawan way.

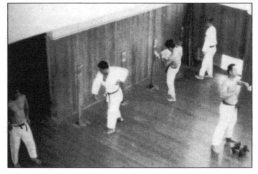

Masaji Taira, 8th *Dan* from the Jundokan *dojo*, faces the *makiwara* daily. The power of his punch is legendary as is the shock delivered by his blocks.

At the Jundokan *dojo* in Naha, Okinawa. The *makiwara* has always played an important role in the student's *karate* education. This photograph was taken in 1973.

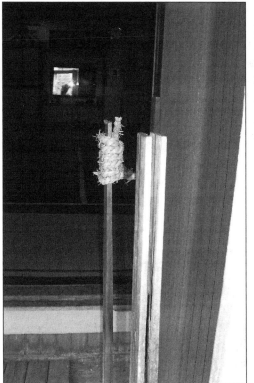

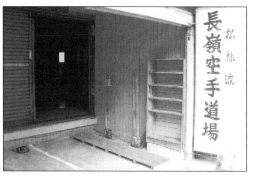

In the entrance to the Kodokan *dojo* in Kume, Okinawa, stand two *makiwara* placed there by the late Shoshin Nagamine. The sign reads, "Shorin ryu, Nagamine Karate Dojo."

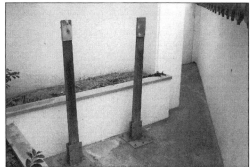

Notice the two different types of *makiwara* at the Kodokan. The tool in the foreground has been deliberately split down most of its length to increase the feeling of resistance.

Just outside the entrance to the Shorinkan *dojo* of Shugoro Nakazato (b. 1921) in Aja, Okinawa, the author found these two *makiwara* tucked away around a corner. Both looked like they were well used.

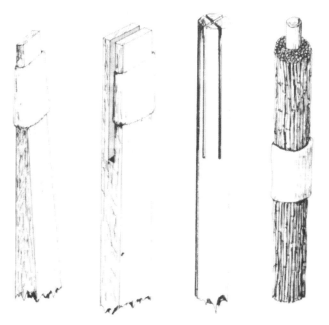

Four different types of *makiwara*, as seen here, allow a large variety of techniques to be worked on and present many opportunities to condition all four limbs.

The *makiwara* is perhaps the most recognizable tool of all those used in *hojo undo* training today, and is one of only a couple the Japanese have used to any degree since beginning their push to absorb Okinawan *karate* into their own home-grown family of martial arts during the early years of the twentieth century. From Japan, *karate* spread worldwide and thus the *makiwara* has traveled with it. Still, this training device in its most recognizable form remains a truly Okinawan innovation.[16] Originally, the name was related to the straw rope used to wrap around the wooden post. The straw was said by some to have had antiseptic properties that were released when the fist pounded it with continuous punches. When the skin of the first two knuckles of each fist began to bruise and even split, the oil in the straw was said to have helped keep the wounds clean. However, this theory is not backed up by personal accounts of people like Hirokazu Kanazawa, Shiro Asano, and Masao Kawasoe, *karateka* who still remember the agony of straw splinters being embedded in their flesh.[17] Regardless of the veracity of such "therapeutic" claims attributed to the use of straw, people were using what they had at hand (no pun intended). These days, most striking pads found on *makiwara* are made of leather and are padded to a greater or lesser degree with materials ranging from industrial grade rubber to coiled springs. Hygiene too is taken more seriously. You should never use a *makiwara* if other people's blood or skin remains deposited on the striking surface. At my *dojo*, the *makiwara*

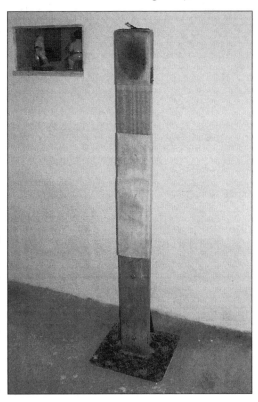

This *makiwara* is in the private *dojo* of Richard Barrett in Almeria, Spain and is typical of the construction methods used when installing a *makiwara* indoors.

is cleaned after every use, regardless of any blood being spilt or skin being lost.

This tool can be freestanding, buried in the earth, or fixed to a wall. The modern portable *makiwara* (of the kind found in martial arts shops around the world) is, in my opinion, so detrimental to the health of the hands that in my mind this type doesn't exist, and no further mention of it will be made. The traditional portable *makiwara,* however, is something entirely different. On Okinawa, two people hold a portable *makiwara* while a third person strikes it. However, because I do not have a portable *makiwara* in my *dojo* and therefore do not train with one on a regular basis, I will not cover its use in this book. Regardless of which type of *makiwara* you face, freestanding, fixed, or portable, it is important to remember the reasons you are standing before it in the first place. The results of continuous training with this tool will leave signs upon the hands, and it has been known for some (immature) people to use the tool solely to achieve those signs. I am of course referring to the set of calloused knuckles found on the person who has become familiar with the *makiwara*. It should be noted that calloused knuckles alone do not indicate the effectiveness of a person's punch. Nor do they speak to his ability as a fighter. They merely register that a lot of impact has occurred between the first two knuckles of the hand and a hard surface. If the tool is used inappropriately or without sincere effort, then, like the use of all the other tools found in *hojo undo*, it will lose any real value for the physical improvement of the person training, or for the development of that person's character. Therefore, you should always use the tool as it was intended to be used. Do not allow a lack of integrity to govern your reason for facing the *makiwara*.

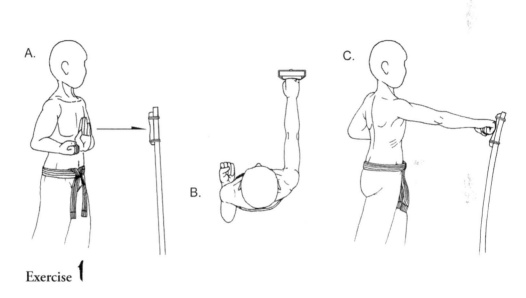

Exercise 1

Stand before the *makiwara* with the left leg slightly forward of the right, with the right arm chambered ready to punch and the left hand beside the punching fist (Figure A). The right hip is lined up with the *makiwara* (Figure B) and the body is held relaxed. With a rotation of the hips and the right arm pulling strongly back across the body to the opposite hip, release the right punch toward the *makiwara* (Figure C). The fist is held tightly and should hit the target with the knuckles of the index and middle fingers only. This keeps the fist in line with the forearm and stops the wrist from buckling on contact with the tool. Inhale before punching and exhale with the punch, the breath and the punch coming to an end at exactly the same time. Return to the starting position and repeat the punch until the appointed number has been reached.

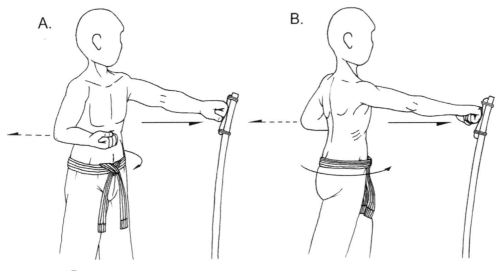

A.   B.

Exercise 2

Standing before the *makiwara* in a natural posture, with the left hip slightly forward, position yourself so that the tool is aligned with the center of the body. From this position throw a punch into the *makiwara* with the left hand (Figure A) and follow this quickly with a strong right punch (Figure B). The combination of punches should be done with a sense of relaxed speed and penetration, the feeling being to hit through the target and not to slow down just before impact is made. In fact, the punch should be accelerating when contact is made and is halted only by the resistance of the *makiwara*. It is this continual battle between the power generated in the punch and the resistance offered by the tool that improves your punching ability over time. Penetration is a vital element of a punch, and nothing is gained by snapping a punch on and off the surface of the tool. The body should support the punches by dropping your weight down slightly and by keeping the back straight and twisting into the punch instead of leaning into it. A strong exhalation too is sometimes used to bring the physical and mental aspect of the technique together. This is *kiai* (*ki*—energy, *ai*—harmony). Though it is not always necessary to take the roof off with a blood-curdling scream when *kiai* is being used, it is, however, necessary to focus the mind, technique, and breath onto one single point in the action. This should be at the point of impact and not a moment too early or too late. The ability to do even this may take some time to acquire. Take it slowly and work patiently toward improving all aspects of punching.

> The term *kiai* (*ki*—your life energy and *ai*—harmony) speaks to the harmony of your mind (intention), your body (the physical technique), your spirit (breath), and the ability to bring all three into focus in the same precise moment. This

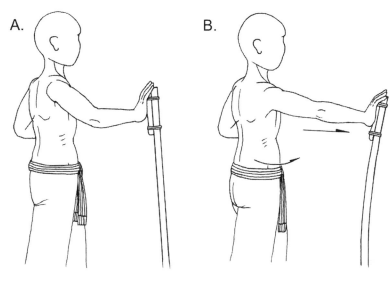

A.   B.

Exercise 3

Stand before the *makiwara* in a natural position with one side slightly forward and the opposite arm held out with the open palm lightly resting on the pad of the tool (Figure A). The other arm is chambered as if ready to punch. Bend the knees a little to lower your body weight and thus the center of gravity. Inhale calmly through the nose. Then with as much explosive power as possible generating from the hips, exhale and thrust the palm into the pad of the *makiwara* (Figure B) as if trying to snap the top off. At first the *makiwara* will no doubt return your energy and spring back just as hard as it was pushed, returning to its normal position without too much effort. Over time, however, it should be made to remain in a bent position for as long as the hand is in contact with the tool. This should not exceed more than a few seconds because the idea of the exercise is to build up a sense of explosive power over a short distance and not to see how long a bent post can be held back. Repeating the exercises on the opposite side ensures an equal progression of ability on both sides of the body. Using the same arm as the forward hip is another way to do this exercise, and all four versions of this exercise should be practiced. It should also be remembered that one side of your body is usually stronger or better coordinated than the other; therefore, more training should be done on the weaker side if you are to even out the progress being made.

has the effect of increasing the sum of the combined parts, making the outcome of the technique far greater than you might imagine. As a concept, *kiai* is found in all Japanese and Okinawan martial arts and is noticeable most often during training by the loud shout issued at the moment a technique is delivered.

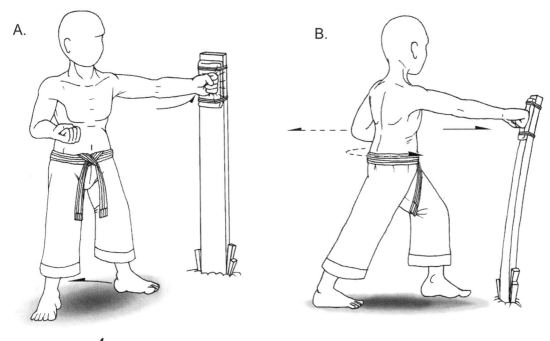

A.

B.

Exercise 4

Standing sideways to the *makiwara* (Figure A), throw an *uraken* (back fist) strike at the target and follow this immediately with a small backward step of the left leg, twisting the body into *zenkutsu dachi* (forward stance). Now facing the *makiwara*, throw a strong *gyaku zuki* punch (Figure B) and *kiai*. Repeat the combination to the desired amount, and then change over to the opposite side. Keep the body relaxed and concentrate on timing, breathing, and gaining a sense of impact.

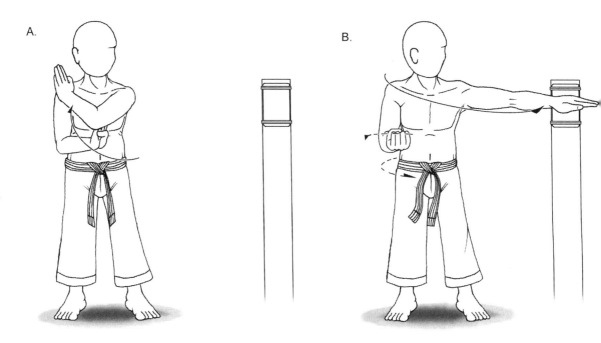

A.

B.

Exercise 5

Standing in a natural posture, with the *makiwara* off to one side, swing the open hand (*shuto uchi*) into the pad when you exhale (Figure A). Withdraw the hand and inhale before striking the tool once more (Figure B). The power behind this technique is generated through the legs and hips, and up through the body, whipping the strike into the *makiwara*. Keep the body in control and make it a part of the strike by employing a good posture and a well-timed sense of focus. The *hekite* (non-striking hand) is withdrawn and chambered on the hip. Again, repeat this exercise with the other hand from the opposite side of the tool.

There are a great many exercises that could be added to this small sample of how to work the *makiwara*, but it was never the intention of this book to cover every exercise that can be done with this or the other tools. To get the most from *hojo undo*, you must learn from a reputable teacher, and then explore for yourself the depth to which you can go with these ancient training methods.

Makiwara Construction Notes

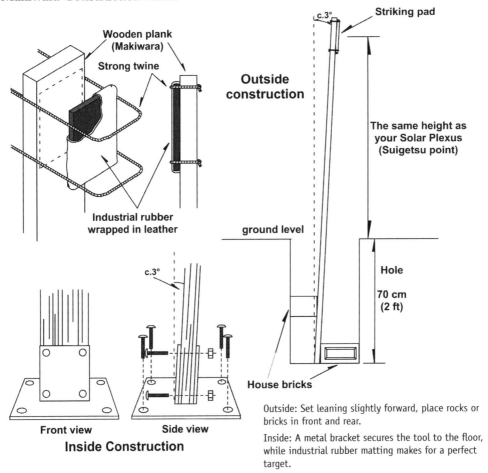

Wooden plank (Makiwara)

Strong twine

Industrial rubber wrapped in leather

Outside construction

c.3°

Striking pad

The same height as your Solar Plexus (Suigetsu point)

ground level

Hole

70 cm (2 ft)

House bricks

c.3°

Front view

Side view

Inside Construction

Outside: Set leaning slightly forward, place rocks or bricks in front and rear.

Inside: A metal bracket secures the tool to the floor, while industrial rubber matting makes for a perfect target.

This tool can be placed either inside or outside the *dojo*. Traditionally it was found standing in backyards throughout the length and breadth of Okinawa and is perhaps the island's one great contribution to the *hojo undo* orchestra. Even men who did not train in *karate* would gather to strike the *makiwara* and test their punching power.[18]

The important thing to remember when making a *makiwara* is that the center of the punching target should be at chest height to correspond with the *suigetsu* point (*solar plexus*) of the person building it, because this is the primary target for the basic *chudan zuki* (mid-level punch) found in *karate* practice.

Outside

A *makiwara* usually measures about four inches (10 cm) in width and is made from hard wood similar to oak. It should be solid but flexible because a *makiwara* with no movement does more harm than good to the *karateka* who uses it. Plant it into a hole in the ground about two feet deep (70 cm); house bricks or large stones are placed in front of the *makiwara* at the bottom of the hole before partly filling it with earth. Just below the surface, more bricks or stones are placed at the back of the *makiwara* before more earth is placed on top to close the hole level with the surrounding surface. The earth should be packed hard around the *makiwara* throughout the "planting," and wooden wedges are often required to complete the process of fixing the tool firmly with the ground. The impact pad is rarely made of straw these days and is more likely to be made of leather. It should not be overly padded! Nevertheless, it should be kept completely free of dirt, blood, or loose skin that may be deposited there during use. The post should lean slightly forward to encourage the index and fore knuckles of the striking fist to make impact on the target and add to the resistance offered by the tool. When not in use, keep the top of the *makiwara* covered and protected from the elements by some kind of hood. A traditional wooden cover is what I use on my *makiwara*.

Inside

When a *makiwara* is placed inside the *dojo,* it is often impossible to excavate a hole in the ground. In such cases, fixing the tool to the ground by means of a strong metal bracket is often the next best option. Again, the height of the target should correspond with the user's chest. The bracket is fixed to the floor with screws and the *makiwara* is then placed securely in the bracket.

As well as the makiwara mentioned above, there are variations of the tool in use by karateka both in Okinawa and around the world. As already mentioned, I do not have a portable makiwara in my dojo and have used this alternative tool only sparingly in the past. However, I am providing a detailed drawing of how to make one and show a photograph of this tool being used in Okinawa. I would again remind those of you who embark on such a project to consider carefully the quality of the materials and method of construction you use. Poorly made tools or low quality materials may produce a 'nice-looking' tool, but such an approach is gambling with safety and runs contrary to the purpose and practice of hojo undo.

An alternative makiwara, made by using a car tire (tyre), offers extra elements to training that are not found when using the more traditional tool; this includes combinations of blocks, strikes, and kicks, coupled with movement of the tool itself. With the alternative makiwara, you will be able to execute techniques in a way approaching a more natural fighting manner. As well as the central target in the middle of the wood, the side of the tire is also struck (and kicked) with various combinations of techniques. For example, push one side of the tire away. The opposite side then swings in and is blocked or checked prior to a counter punch being thrown into the target. A slight adjustment in distance from the tool allows for kicks to be used too. In order to achieve this movement, hang the tool from a post or against a pillar of a wall, as seen in the photo taken at the Higaonna dojo in Kiyose, Tokyo. Should you wish to use it as a traditional makiwara, place it against a flat wall that is strong enough to take the repeated force of the impact.

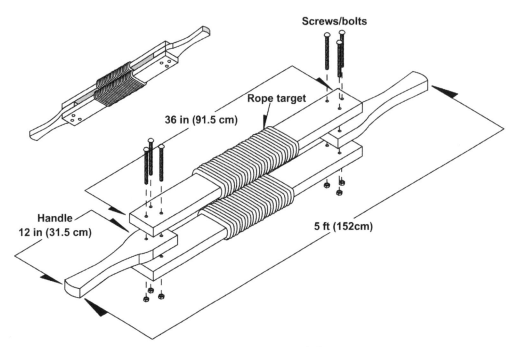

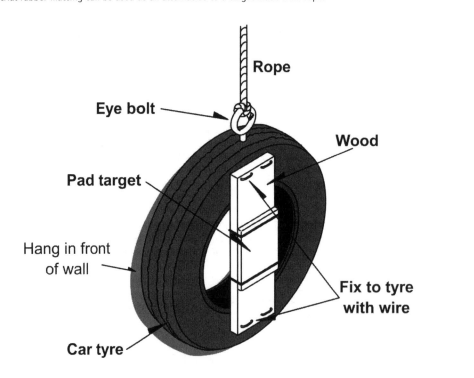

Screws/bolts

Rope target

36 in (91.5 cm)

Handle
12 in (31.5 cm)

5 ft (152cm)

Industrial rubber matting can be used as an alternative to a target made from rope.

Rope

Eye bolt

Wood

Pad target

Hang in front
of wall

Fix to tyre
with wire

Car tyre

Hung against a tree trunk or internal pillar, this tool allows for blocking and punching combinations to be practiced.

Tou – Bamboo Bundle

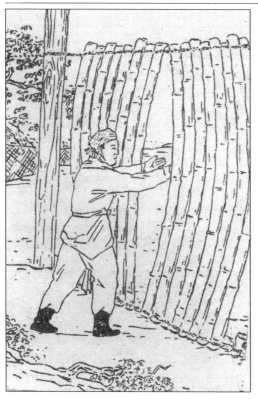

As this old drawing shows, pushing the hands through lengths of bamboo to condition the fingers is nothing new.

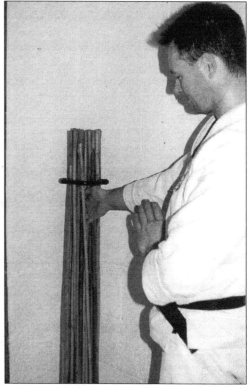

Taken in the mid-1980's, this photograph shows Richard Barrett training with the *tou*.

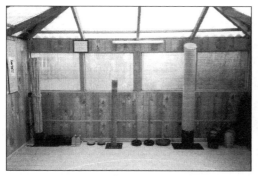

Before relocating to Spain, Richard Barrett *sensei* built a small *dojo* behind his home in Hertfordshire where he trained himself as well as a small group of students. *Hojo undo* played an important role in all of the training.

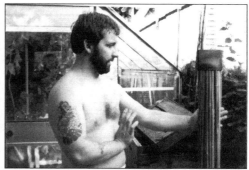

The author was first introduced to the *tou* by Richard Barrett. This photograph was taken during his first encounter with the tool. It hurt!

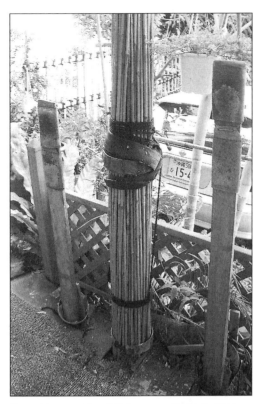

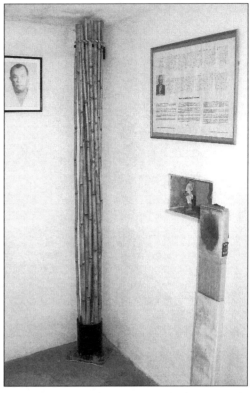

The *makiwara* and *tou* at Hokama *sensei*'s *dojo* in Nishi-hara, Okinawa stand to one side of the entrance and are used often by the students who train there.

At his private *dojo* in Almeria, Spain, Richard Barrett con-tinues to train himself in the traditional Okinawan way. The *makiwara* and *tou* are just two of the tools he uses.

When you take into account the number of times the technique *nukite* (spear hand) is used in *karate kata*, it should come as no surprise to learn that there exists a training tool to facilitate the growth of strong fingertips within the *hojo undo* arsenal. In fact, a number of tools survive that center on the development of the fingers, some of which you will find within the pages of this book. However the *tou*, sometimes called *taketaba*, is perhaps one of the best-suited tools for allowing the *karateka* to feel the impact of their spear-hand strikes in a way that closely resembles the situation in which such a strike would most likely be deployed. Standing in a fighting posture, upright and within reach of the *tou,* it is possible to thrust the hand into the tool and withdraw it again before moving swiftly to the side and making a second strike. Grasping the bundle, too, can be done from many angles including a kneeling posture that simulates an attack to the inside of the legs or groin area.

I have been unable to discover the singular origin for this particular tool. Opinions vary, although from old Chinese drawings it is clear that such a tool or something very similar has been in use for centuries. Whether or not the Okinawans took their inspiration for the *tou* directly from such martial arts texts as they could find in China[19] or developed it themselves through the use or cultivation of the native vegetation, I cannot say for sure. Nevertheless, it is not beyond the realm of possibility to imagine the Okinawans using recently harvested bundles of sugar cane or the reeds they used for their thatched roofs to test their techniques. Such activities could have led to the birth of the *tou*. This is speculation on my part, true, but not an altogether unreasonable hypothesis when you understand the ingenuity of the Okinawan people and their highly developed sense of adapting things to suit their needs. Its simple construction and easy-to-find materials have always made the *tou* one of the easiest tools to acquire, if not to use. With perseverance, the *tou* helps those who wish to develop their *nukite* strike into a technique that is both simple in its execution and yet shocking to the recipient. It seems to me an overly simplistic approach to *karate* to practice techniques in *kata* that cannot be utilized should the need arise. The name *nukite* (spear hand) speaks to the nature of the technique, and who among us would choose to go into battle with a plastic spear? Just as fighting men of olden times kept their swords sharp and modern day solders keep their firearms clean, I believe today's *karateka* are obliged to equip themselves with bodies, minds, and techniques that are capable of living up to the purpose of *karate*, and that is to increase the odds in our favor should we ever be attacked. To do otherwise is a bit like owning a Ferrari without the engine; it looks good, but is of little value except as an ornament.

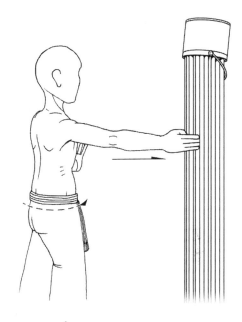

Exercise 1

Stand at arm's length and thrust a hand into the bundle using the *nukite* technique. Take care to hold the fingers as tightly together as possible and try not to let them separate when the hand penetrates the tool. Make sure the thumb is tucked in hard against the side of the hand. Like the punch, make full use of the opposite, returning hand (*hekite*) when practicing. Remember to breathe in first and to exhale with the strike.

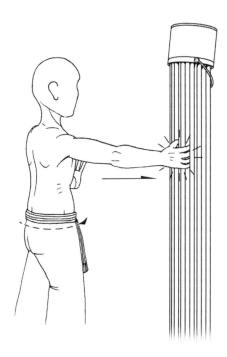

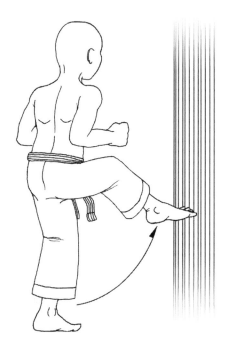

Exercise 2

A powerful gripping action can be acquired simply by grabbing at the bundle from the outside and giving it a slight pull while closing the armpit down before releasing it, and then grabbing it with the opposite hand. After one or two grabs like this, begin to move around the tool, all the while remembering to alter the height of the strike upon the *tou* as you do so. In a real confrontation, it would be a mistake to aim all your blows at one spot on the opponent's body; therefore, moving around the *tou* and varying the target keeps the practice that one step closer to reality.

Exercise 3

A favorite of *karateka* from the *Pangai Noon ryu, Uechi ryu,* and *Shohei ryu* schools of Okinawan *karatedo* is to use the *tou* in much the same way as a heavy kick bag might be used. In these schools of *karate,* the practitioners make a point of kicking with the tips of the toes, giving them an opportunity to work on penetrating the target. It is also helpful when impacting with the *koshi* (hard pad on the foot at the base of the toes), the more usual foot position used in most *karate* traditions. Either technique will be helped by constant repetition, and in this simple truth lays the "secret" of improvement.

Tou Construction Notes

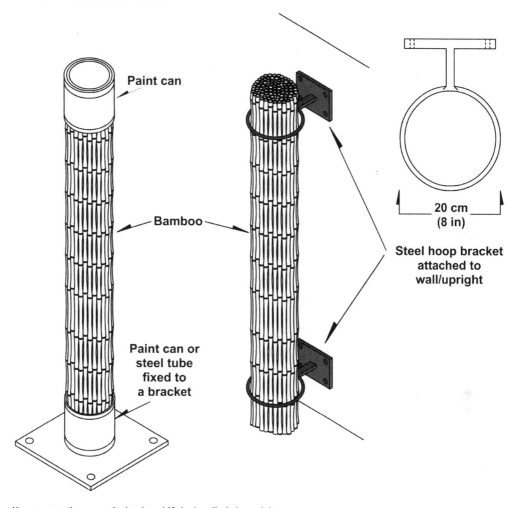

Paint can

Bamboo

Paint can or steel tube fixed to a bracket

Steel hoop bracket attached to wall/upright

20 cm (8 in)

More penetrative power is developed if the bundle is kept tight.

Perhaps the easiest of tools to build, the *tou* can be made from a bunch of bamboo garden stakes and two old paint cans, one placed on either end of the bundle. The tool can be fixed to the ground with a bracket made from an old paint can or short length of steel tubing. A pair of steel wall brackets (similar to small basketball hoops) can also be used placed one above the other with the bamboo simply stacked loosely between the two.

Jari Bako – Sand Box

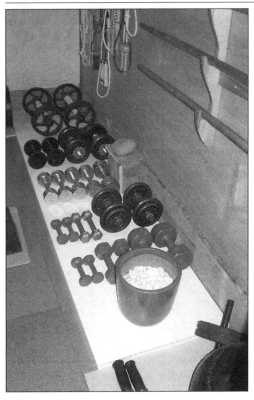

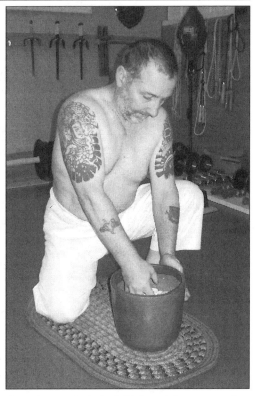

Jari bako and a small number of the weights and tools used at the author's Shinseidokan *dojo* in Tasmania.

The author uses both the *jari bako* and the *tou* to condition his fingers and afford him an effective *nukite* (spear hand) strike.

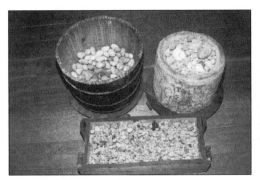

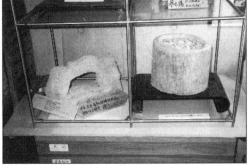

These *jari bako*, sometimes called '*suna bako*' or '*kan shu*', from times gone by are on display at the Okinawa Karate Museum.

Ancient *ishisashi* and *jari bako* on display at the Okinawa Karate Museum in Nishihara.

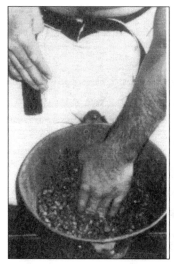 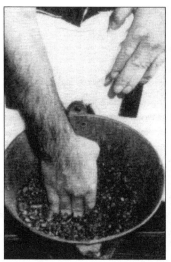 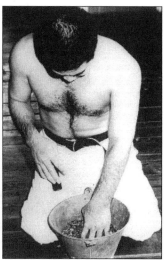

As with the *makiwara*, both hands are conditioned, but not equally. The least prominent hand, the left if you are right handed, should be used more until it begins to feel as strong as the prominent hand.

Thrusting the fingers into gravel conditions them to the impact encountered when thrusting into a soft target on a body

A photograph of Morio Higaonna training with the *jari bako* at the Yoyogi *dojo* in Tokyo during the 1970s.

A very simple training aid to construct, but make no mistake about it, it will test your resolve. Basically made from a box, a bucket, or a container of almost any kind, and filled with either sand or small stones, this is what Gichin Funakoshi, the founder of the *Shotokan karate* tradition had to say about it:

> *While there is no escaping the brutal makiwara, there are numerous other ways karate jutsu uses to condition the body. For example, training the fingers so that one is capable of piercing or pressing them into the weak parts of the body requires filling a container with sand so that repeated thrusting into it helps develop and harden the tips of your fingers.* (p. 26)

However, this is what another famous Okinawan *karate sensei* (teacher), Kinjo Hiroshi, a student of Chojo Oshiro and later, Chomo Hanashiro, had to say on the subject of hand conditioning in a conversation with Charles Radi:

> *I don't believe karate anywhere in the world today is the same as it was during the old days in Okinawa. There are several reasons why I believe this and one of them is simply because so much has been handed down incorrectly. One example is hand conditioning; some believe that by thrusting your hand into a box filled with sand, or into a bundle of bamboo, your fingertips will be hardened and better prepared to use as a weapon. This is not true and people who employ such training methods are liable to irreparably injure*

themselves and not continue with karate. Makiwara (of which there are several kinds) has long been the accepted apparatus for developing your hands and impact-related skills. [20]

While both of these great teachers of *karate* come from a similar background and *karate* tradition (*Shuri-te*), they are a few generations apart, with Mr. Funakoshi (now deceased) being the older. Clearly, they hold different opinions about the value of certain pieces of equipment used in *hojo undo*. This raises an interesting point: do we need to use all the tools and methods that fall under the banner of *hojo undo* or simply utilize those tools and training drills that we find of benefit to us? The purpose of this book is to introduce a variety of tools and training drills and to allow you, the reader, to form your own opinion about whether such training will enhance your *karate*, or not!

Within the *Naha-te* tradition of *karate* on Okinawa (*Goju ryu, Uechi ryu,* etc.), conditioning has always played a more dominant role in the overall training undergone by students than in those schools of *karate* that evolved from *Shuri-te* and *Tomari-te*. Nevertheless, this should not be interpreted as being either better or worse; it is merely a difference of approach to answering the same age-old question: "How do I best prepare to defend myself?" For me, training with these tools over the years has provided an opportunity to test my mental resolve and my physical endurance, and to gain an understanding of where my limits lie in each. Because of this, I know for sure my weak points and my strengths, and for me this provides a great advantage over people who think they know theirs. *Hojo undo* training is not about how many tools we use or how good we look using them; it is about being honest in our efforts and honest with ourselves, and reaping the rewards inherent in both.

At first, the container being used as a *jari bako* should be filled some way to the top with rough sand. Later on, this can be replaced with small pebbles. Discretion is required here and your ability to continue using this tool should be at the forefront of your mind when choosing the kind of material with which to fill the container. For example, rough sand or beads can be used, or it may be that you might begin training with softer (builder's) sand before replacing it with gravel or moving on to small stones.

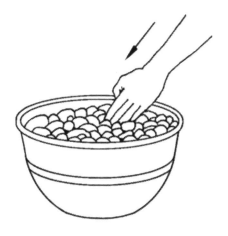

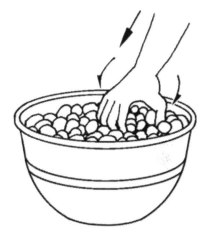

Exercise 1

By placing the container on a low table or ledge, it is possible to drop into *shiko dachi* and thrust the fingertips into the contents using *nukite* (spear hand). If this is not possible, simply place the container on the floor, position yourself comfortably, and do the exercises from there. Effort should be focused on making the tips of the fingers acclimatized to impact, so ease up on the idea of penetrating as deeply as you can. Over time, you will feel you can go a little deeper, and this is the time to make an effort. You can also try bending the middle finger slightly to allow the tip of it, and those of the fingers on either side, to become level. Squeeze the tips of all three fingers tightly together and use this hand formation in the same way as *nukite*.

Exercise 2

As with the *tou*, the practice can be changed to introduce a grabbing action, although it is not necessary to pull here. Just open the hand and thrusting the fingers into the container, make a grabbing action before withdrawing the hand. Whatever method is used, it is important to train in accordance with your abilities and slowly try to push the boundaries of those abilities. Remember to inhale and then make a powerful exhalation with each thrust of the hand. Patience is required to make progress with *hojo undo*: patience and perseverance. It is not important to do fifty strikes on your first attempt. As always in *karate* training, we are aspiring for quality over quantity. It is the quality of the blows that are important, and not necessarily the number.

Perhaps this is also an opportune time to dispel some of the well-established myths and legends surrounding the use of your bare hands. As mentioned at the beginning of this book, Okinawa is a treasure trove of stories and folklore surrounding the exploits of martial artists of long ago. Again, I have to say that many of these stories have to be taken with a large pinch of salt. Nevertheless, they serve an important function, in my opinion, and that is the feeling of inspiration they can offer us, the present generation of *karateka*.

For as long as I can remember I have heard stories about the founder of *Goju ryu karate*, Chojun Miyagi, and how he could, and did, tear strips of meat off a side of beef with nothing but his fingers. Another tale tells of how he could clench a bamboo shaft and crush it with his grip. Well, he is no longer alive to say, one way or the other, and I am not suggesting for a moment that the strength of his grip was not indeed tremendous; in fact, I have met and trained with six of Chojun Miyagi's direct students[21] and received first-hand accounts to confirm that he did possess a very powerful grip. However, everything I know about the man leads me to believe that he would have avoided such public displays of strength. I am left thinking that perhaps such exploits arose from the minds of his followers and admirers who, innocently enough, bestowed upon Mr. Miyagi abilities he may not have had. Alternatively, perhaps they just exaggerated things a little? Almost identical tales have been told about other past *karate* masters, such as Gichin Funakoshi's teachers, Itosu and Azato for example. Both men were considered among the finest karate men of their time in Okinawa. Of Itosu he said: "Renowned for his grip strength, my own teacher, Itosu Anko, once broke a 15 cm length of bamboo into three or four pieces as requested." And of Azato, his other teacher, he said: "A master of *nukite* (spear hand) Azato *sensei* was well known for his strength and powerful fingers. Once, as an adolescent, he went to the local slaughterhouse and drove his fingers into the lifeless body of a pig using this technique." (p. 64)

It all sounds very familiar, does it not? But no matter, for as I have previously pointed out, such tales abound on Okinawa, and whether there may be some reality-based truth to these stories or not, their value today lies in their ability to inspire and enthuse the imagination of others, a gift left to us from long ago that many leave unused and unvalued. How short-sighted!

Jari Bako Construction Notes

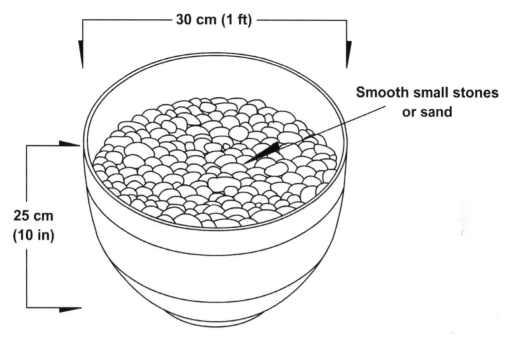

30 cm (1 ft)

Smooth small stones
or sand

25 cm
(10 in)

Round stones or rough sand help develop strong fingertips.

Almost any container can serve to make this tool, as long as it is made of material sufficient to take the punishment of frequent use and is wide enough to allow movement of the sand or stones when the fingers penetrate the contents. Smooth, marble-sized stones or, indeed, marbles themselves can be used though some people prefer to use rough sand or gravel to thrust their fingers into. Whatever material is used, anything with sharp edges should always be avoided.

Ude Kitae – Pounding Post

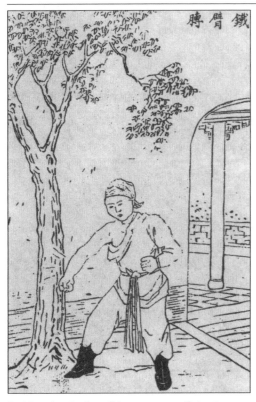

In this early print from China, we can see that nature provided the tools to work with. Here a small tree is used as an *ude kitae*.

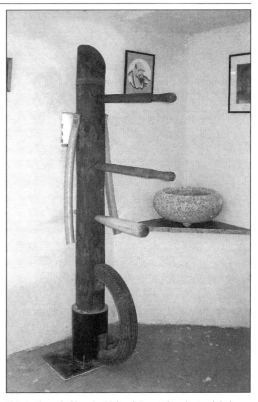

This is the *ude kitae* in Richard Barrett's private *dojo* in Almeria, Spain. Note the arms and 'leg' made from half a motorcycle tire. The three wooden arms can be set in any number of combinations or removed altogether.

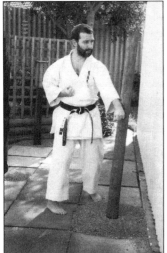

An understanding of all the basic blocks, such as this *gedan barai*, is enhanced by working with the *ude kitae*.

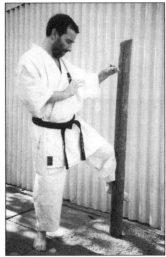

Continuous tapping is the key here, not full power kicking. The author is seen here working on his legs back in 1996 at the age of 41.

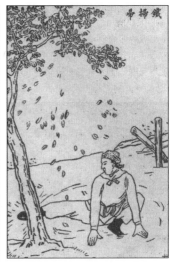

Against the legs too, a small tree can be a great training partner.

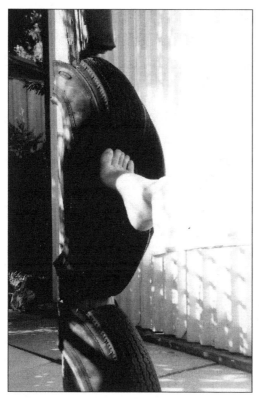

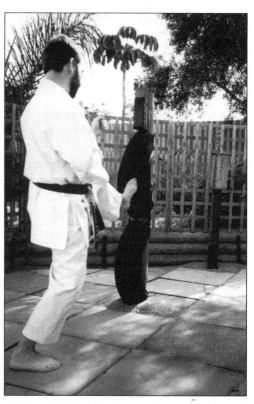

Car tires offer good resistance and allow a feeling of penetration when punching, kicking, or striking. Without this feeling, there is a danger of hitting to the target instead of through it. In a real situation, the difference could prove costly. Because the body tends to do what we train it to do, knowing what we are capable of is a valuable asset.

Ude kitae with tires helps develop the hips and the use of *koshi*, thrusting the hips.

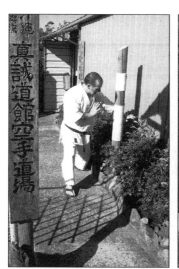

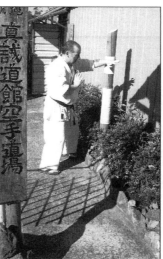

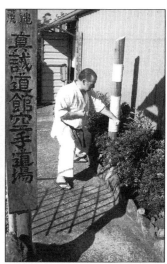

Twelve years, and countless strikes on the *ude kitae*, separate this photograph from those taken in the author's *dojo* in Western Australia. With *hojo undo*, as with all martial arts, it is important to continue once you start.

Strikes too, like this *shuto uchi* (knife hand strike) can be worked on the *ude kitae*.

Even basic blocking, like this *gedan barai* (low swinging block), takes on a whole new 'feeling' when done with intent against an unforgiving training partner like the *ude kitae*.

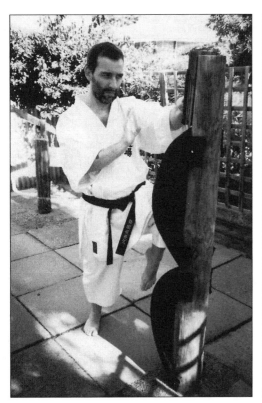
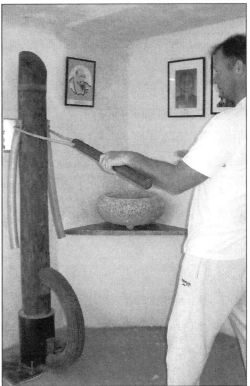

Exploding forward into the *ude kitae* with a combination of a knee kick, *heiza geri*, followed immediately by a punch to the face, *jodan zuki* allows the generation of maximum force—something that just cannot be practiced on a training partner.

Richard Barrett training with the *ude kitae*. With this set up, he has to maintain a pulling action on the wooden arm prior to kicking. The arm on a rope is also used to practice the *hikei uke* (grasping block) combination found in a number of *Goju ryu kata*.

Set the post in the ground firmly enough to allow very little movement. The *ude kite* post is used to condition the hands, arms, legs, and feet. This tool comes in many forms, and when building one, the height and diameter of the wooden post being used should be taken into account according to how you intend to use it. Too slim and it cannot stand up to the pounding it receives; too big, and it may have no "give" in it at all. Neither of these allows the tool to be used as intended. With regard to height, at least head height is recommended, or even a little taller. If the tip of the post is cut off at an angle, it allows the *tettsui uchi* (hammer fist) technique to be practiced. Take care to start slowly, and build up the level of impact you can make and take over a number of months. Every blocking action found in *karate* can be trained with the *ude kitae*, as can the striking and thrusting techniques. Conditioning the lower leg as well as the arms in time provides the *karateka* with a "third limb" when sitting in *nekoashi dachi* (cat stance) with which to

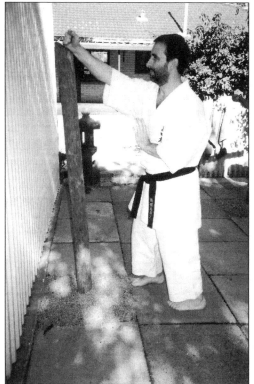

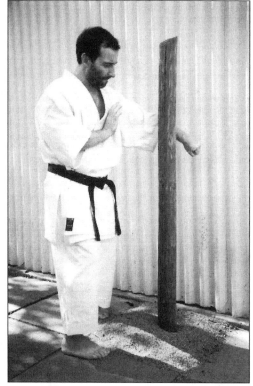

Forging the techniques found in the *kata*, the value of *hojo undo* training becomes apparent.

The inside of the arm is often used to block and should not be neglected. Here the author blocks on an inward swing.

defend against kicks. This is particularly useful because it frees the *karateka* from dropping his arms when dealing with a low (*gedan*) attack.

Although often a far simpler tool in construction to that of its Chinese predecessor, the Okinawan *ude kitae* is no less helpful in its ability to toughen up the limbs and the minds of those who use it. The "wooden-man," also known as *Mook Jung* or *Muk Yang Jong* found in Chinese schools of combat from *Shaolin* boxing to *Wing-Chun kung-fu* since ancient times has, as standard, arms and even a leg with which to target your blows, whereas the *ude kitae* on Okinawa tends to be a far more simple piece of equipment. Still, this has not stopped enterprising *karateka* over the years from improvising to fashion the tool into a training partner upon whom they can employ the full range of techniques from their own personal repertoire.

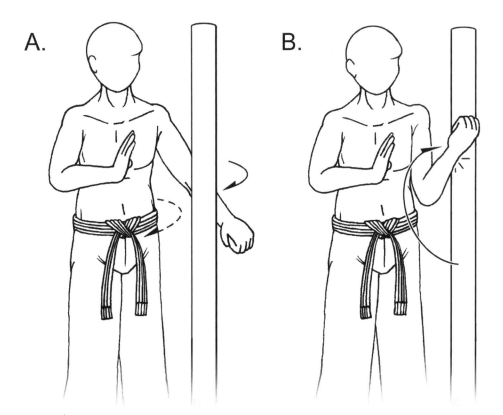

A.

B.

Exercise 1

Stand before the tool and execute the basic blocks in a flowing, rhythmical way, moving from *gedan barai* (low swinging block, Figure A) up to *chudan uchi uke* (mid-level block, Figure B) before changing arms. This exercise can be lengthened by adding more blocks and by moving around the tool and switching from outside to inside blocks.

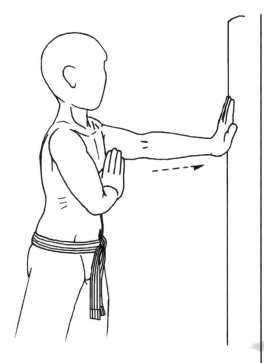

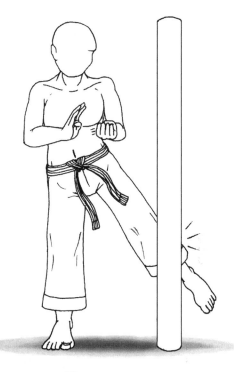

Exercise 2

Shotei uchi (palm heel strike) can be practiced from any number of stances. A variation of this strike would be to stand with the palm already resting lightly against the tool; then with a sharp thrust of the hip, push into the post as if to uproot it from the ground. This is similar to the thrusting exercise done with the *makiwara*.

Exercise 3

Standing on one leg, use the post to condition the shins and legs by "tapping" it over and over again until that particular part of the body becomes resistant to the impact of a blow. In between conditioning the shins, the practice of *ashi barai* (leg sweep) allows the training of the legs to continue while the shins get a rest.

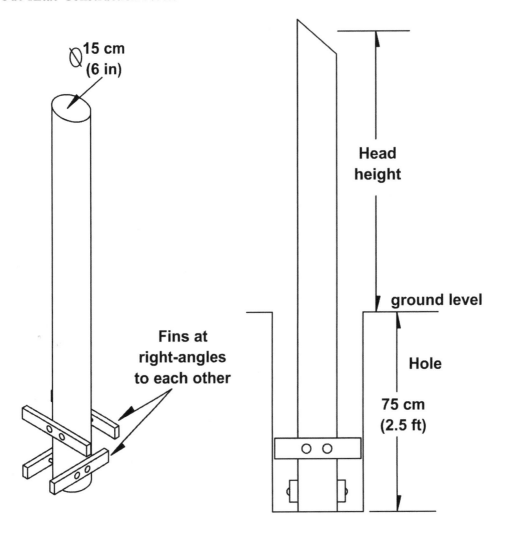

15 cm
(6 in)

Fins at
right-angles
to each other

Head
height

ground level

Hole

75 cm
(2.5 ft)

Angle the top to increase the variety of strikes one can practice.

You need a round fence post, or the sort of garden landscaping post that can be purchased from plant nurseries or the larger hardware outlets. It must be long enough to bury at least twenty-four inches (61 cm) of it in the ground and still have it stand at head height. Before burying the post, attach fins to the bottom to help with its stability once training commences. Setting the fins in cement may be advisable if the tool is being used in sandy soil. Alternatively, set the post in a bracket made from industrial tubing and fix the bracket to a concrete path, driveway, or *dojo* floor with strong bolts.

Kakite Bikei – Blocking Post

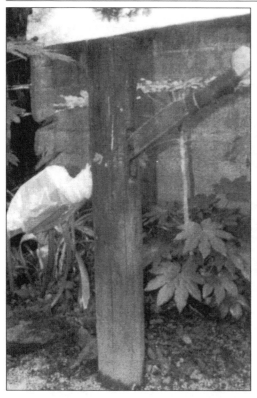

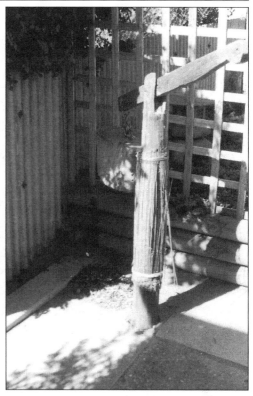

This photo appeared in the *Karate-do* magazine (Japan) in 2003 and was used by a practitioner of the Okinawan system of *karate*, *To-on ryu*.

The author's *kakite bikei* stood outside his *dojo* for eight years and was used almost every day.

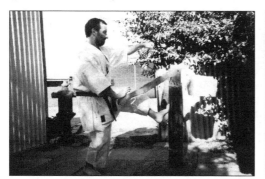

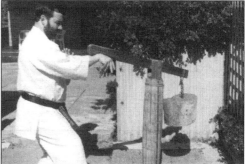

Kicks too can be used as shown here, off the front leg.

The author training at his *dojo* in Perth, Western Australia, 1996.

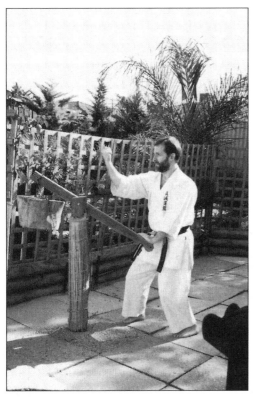

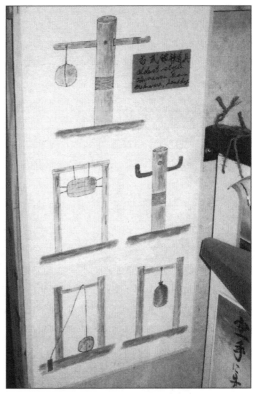

Pushing the attacking arm down and delivering a rolling back fist strike to the face is a combination found in many martial arts.

These drawings, on display at the Okinawa Karate Museum in Nishihara, show an array of different tools used by Okinawan *karateka* to condition their bodies.

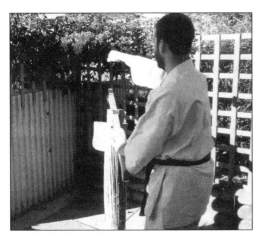

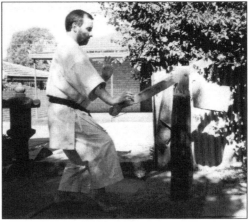

In addition to blocking, defensive and offensive combinations can also be practiced.

All the blocks found in *karate* can be practiced on this tool.

Finding this training tool is rare these days, although this fact alone should not stop anybody from constructing one. In thirty-five years of *karate* training, I have never come across one in Okinawa, nor in any *dojo* apart from my own. Drawings and early photographs often show the arm fixed to the side of the upright post and held there with a single bolt. Nevertheless, I found this method of construction to be less successful than having the arm of the tool sit in a groove cut down the center of the post. In October 1996, when Hirokazu Kanazawa *sensei*, head of the Shotokan Karatedo International Federation, visited my home, he was fascinated by the tools standing in the small courtyard next to my *dojo*.[22] He took time out to train on the *makiwara* and the two types of *ude kitae*, but was unsure of how to use the *kakite bikei*. Being the kind of man he is, however, he wasted no time soliciting information from me on just how it was done. This I took as a sign of the great man's complete lack of ego, and it was an honor for me to pass on to him what little information I could give him about the tool.

A post set in the ground with a "key" cut out at the top through which a bolt is passed, holding a wooden arm that is counterbalanced by a weight, and a pad wrapped around the post that allows kicking to be practiced make the *kakite bikei* a particularly good tool for working on blocking and kicking combinations. Even though the tool itself cannot move (apart from the arm), the *karateka* can and should move around it, executing their techniques from different angles and distances. These can be simple one-block techniques or combinations involving grabs and kicks. However, the real value derived from this tool lies in your ability to move around it while blocking, gripping, and striking in as many different ways as possible. This tool challenges your perception of *ma ai* (distance) and focus. The *kakite bikei* is, in common with all the other tools found in *hojo undo*, a hard training partner that is unforgiving of mistakes and takes all you can give and stand ready for more. Deciding on a number of techniques or a length of time to spend working on the tool, and then sticking with it, tests the user considerably. As time goes by, increase the number of techniques or the length of time.

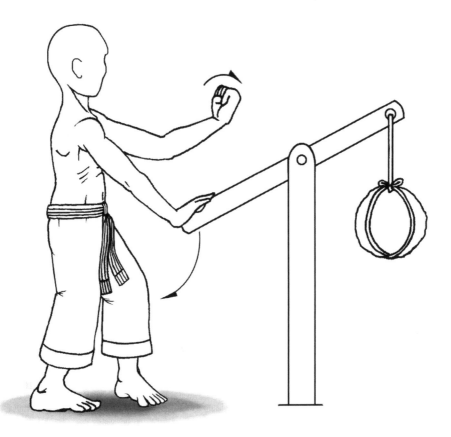

Exercise 1

A *shotei uke* (pressing block) and a *uraken* (back fist strike) is a combination that can be practiced while moving in and back, controlling the arm of the tool while you do so. Switching over and over from left to right adds to the strength of this exercise, and I would encourage users to work the tool until exhausted.

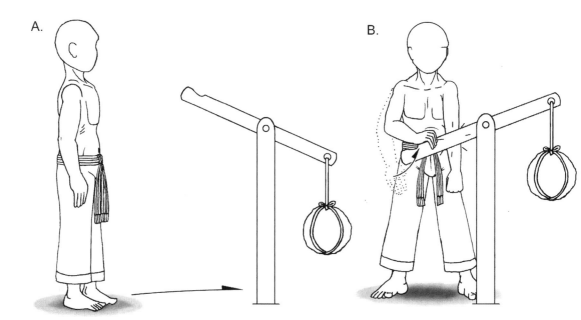

A.

B.

Exercise 2

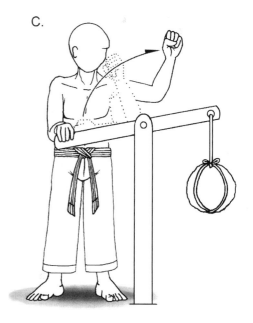

C.

Stand in front of the tool (Figure A) and using *tai sabaki* (body shifting), quickly shift to the left of the arm, blocking the limb of the tool with a left forearm *furi uke* (swinging block) while at the same time gripping the arm of the tool with the right hand (Figure B); continue on to perform *jodan hidari tettsui uchi* (left-side hammer-fist strike to the head, Figure C). This exercise emulates the opening sequence from the *Goju ryu kata saifa* and the *Shotokan kata chinte*. Again, moving in from the left and then from the right of the tool helps to develop skills such as entering (*irimi*) and switching sides smoothly and quickly (*hantai*). It also improves your stamina and encourages the examination of your breathing patterns. Remember, if our breath is not working with us then it is working against us, for there is no neutral position when it comes to our bodies' physical exertion and the energy-giving properties of our breath.

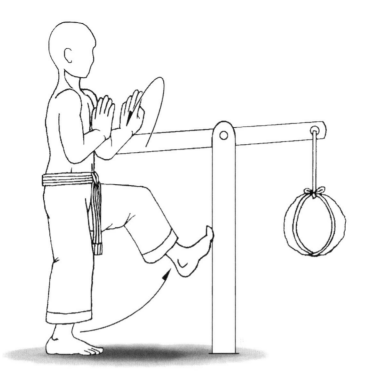

Exercise 3

Hikei uke (grasping block) and *mae geri* (front kick) combined with the switching from side to side that this tool encourages is a good way to develop a sense of rhythm. Remembering to keep the armpit closed when blocking and keeping your balance are just two of the things to work on when training with this exercise.

Kakite Bikei Construction Notes

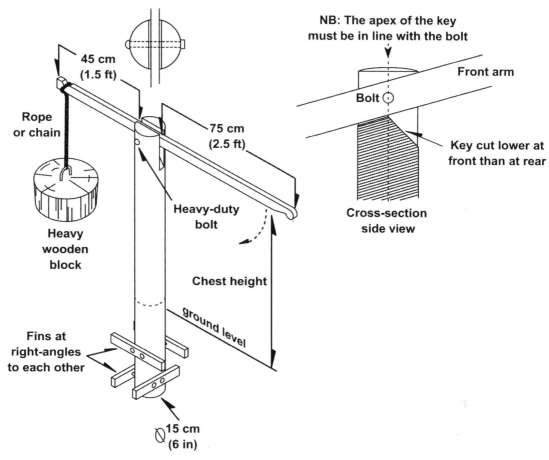

Add fins to increase stability, and a counterweight heavy enough to offer a challenge to the user.

Like the *ude kitae*, this tool should have fins fitted to the base of the post before being buried in the earth. A key is cut in the center of the top of the post and holes drilled through the remaining sides. A corresponding hole is drilled through the arm at one end of which is fixed a weight sufficient to keep the arm up. It should also be heavy enough to offer serious resistance when the arm is being pushed downward during training. The arm should be built strong enough to withstand the impact of continuous blocking without breaking or the tool twisting in the ground. As with all the tools that are planted in the ground, time should be given to allow them to "settle" once they have been built. Make sure that the earth around the upright has been packed as tightly as possible. If the ground is particularly sandy, pouring cement into the hole around the fins helps with stability. The arm may have to be replaced from time to time, due to the damage imposed on it by the impact of regular training, but like replacing the *makiwara* from time to time, this should be considered normal.

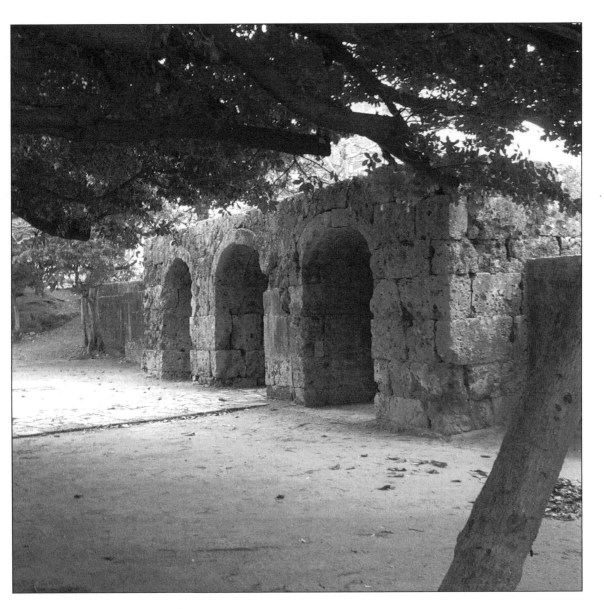

Remains of the gateway to Sogenji temple.

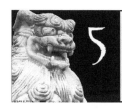

5 BODY CONDITIONING EXERCISES

Ude Tanren – Two-Person Conditioning Exercises

Within the various schools of *karate* in Okinawa, there are also a great many conditioning exercises that are done without tools, but with a training partner instead. To cover all of them and do justice to their value would require a book of its own and is something I am working on. For this reason, only a few *ude tanren* drills have been included here. However, once this kind of training becomes "normal," the variety and combination of strikes and blocks a *karateka* can come up with indicates the progress he is making in the pursuit of realistic impact training for the body and mind. As well as the conditioning of the arms through regular practice, the purpose of *ude tanren* training is to cultivate the ability to deliver and receive "shock," an important element of any *karate* technique, and the very thing that often brings many "thin-air" *karateka* (those who train without making contact with either each other or an appropriate training aid) to a standstill. Much like the drills used against the *ude kitae*, the *ude tanren* exercises encourage the body to condition itself while the mind (attitude) is toughened to withstand

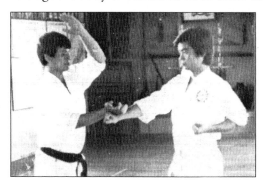

A rare image of training at the *Uechi ryu* headquarters in Okinawa, c. 1970.

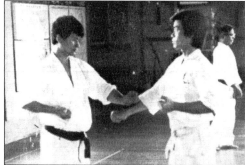

Kanei Uechi *sensei* (in the background) watches over others training, while in the foreground students practice *ude tanren*.

higher levels of discomfort brought on by the shock of collision. With the familiarity of contact comes a kind of reference point in the mind that allows an impact to cause less confusion, in turn, allowing us to continue on to a conclusion. When unfamiliar things happen, our mind automatically tries to work it out. *Ude tanren* familiarizes the mind with close contact and the effects of impact upon the body. In a real situation, it is unreasonable to expect to walk away from a physical altercation without being hit, and for

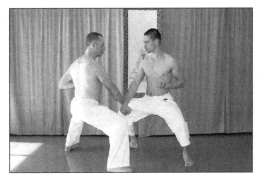

Students at the Shinseidokan *dojo* use *ude tanren* to condition their arms.

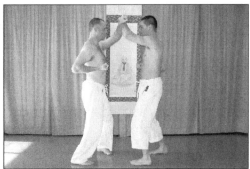

Stepping forward into a block is often a new experience for *karate* students. Most step back when blocking.

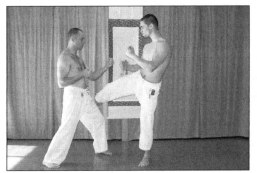

Becoming accustomed to impact on the legs.

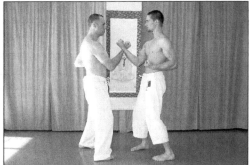

Stepping forward while blocking allows the mind to stay on the offensive.

this reason alone, it is essential that *karateka* work with a training partner (or with tools) on a regular basis, and certainly more often than they work in thin air. *Karate* is an art of self-defense, a martial art, an art that requires not only an ability to hit, but also an ability to withstand being hit. The weakest part of the body is quite often the mind, and *hojo undo* is a well-established method of developing and strengthening it.

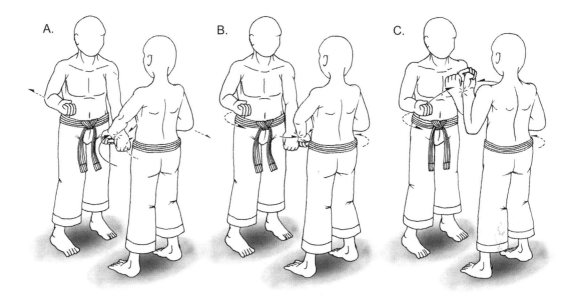

Exercise 1

Begin by facing your training partner and both swing your left arms together in a relaxed manner (Figure A). Impact should be on the inside edge of the arms and not on the soft underside where the veins and arteries are located close to the surface. The aim is to build up the level of acceptable impact, which means heavy contact at an early stage can be counterproductive. Remember to keep the shoulders relaxed and to move with a smooth swinging action. Build from the single impact exercise of an inside (of the arm) *gedan barai*, by continuing through and then swinging the same arm back to make an outside *gedan barai* (Figure B). The training can be built upon even more by combining an inside, and later, an outside *chudan uke* to the practice in a continuous flowing action (Figure C), alternating from arm to arm.

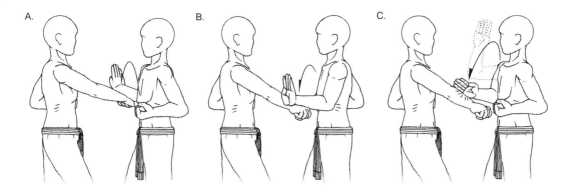

A.　　　　　　　　B.　　　　　　　　C.

Exercise *2*

Other methods of *ude tanren* include stepping forward and backward with a partner while blocking and striking your partner's arm. To achieve this, have one person step forward on the right leg and throw a *chudan zuki* (mid-level punch) with the right hand. At the same time, the other person steps backward with the left leg and blocks with his right hand, using *chudan hikei uke* (mid-level open-hand block, Figure A). Then he repeats the block with the left hand (Figure B) before striking the punching arm with a right-handed *shuto uchi* (open-hand strike, Figure C). At that point the roles are reversed and the defender steps forward with a right-handed *chudan zuki* of his own, while the other person steps backward and repeats the same block and strike combination. This stepping forward and backward can be repeated until the required number has been completed or can be done continually for a set period of time.

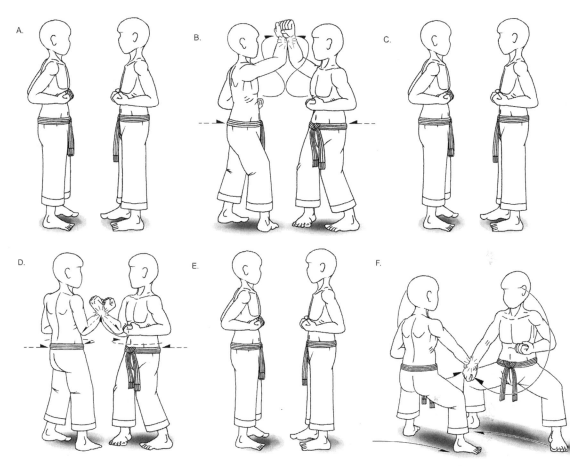

Shodan Uke Barai – One-Step Blocking Practice

Facing your partner and standing in *heiko dachi* (natural stance) about one meter apart (Figure A), both step forward with the right leg into *sanchin dachi*. Immediately after the stance is made, both block with a right *jodan age uke* (high rising block) making impact at the wrist end of the forearm (Figure B). The block is then withdrawn while both step back into *heiko dachi* (Figure C). Repeating this exercise on the right-hand side in quick succession allows a sense of rhythm to be built into the practice and assists with learning how to manage the breath. Exhaling with the block and inhaling while you move back regulates the pace and intensity of the training and stops you from training with excessive speed. After blocking with *jodan* and stepping back, repeat the same exercise with *chudan uke* (mid-level block, Figure D), step back (Figure E) and then forward again with *gedan uke* (lower-level block, Figure F). With the *gedan uke*, step forward into *shiko dachi* (low stance).

A second way to work this drill is to alternate on each count. Begin with a left step forward into *sanchin dachi*, left *jodan uke*; step back. Then right step forward, right *chudan uke*; step back. Follow by a left step forward into *shiko dachi*, left *gedan barai*, before stepping back for a third time. Once this can be done with control, expand the exercise further by continuing to change over and over until the desired number of repetitions has been completed or a set time has elapsed.

Sandan Uke Barai – Three-Step Blocking Practice

Also known by the name *san dan gi* (three-step technique), this practice introduces consecutive forward and backward stepping. Begin by standing about one meter apart from your training partner (Figure A). One person steps forward with the right leg into *sanchin dachi* and punches *jodan zuki* (head high punch) with the right hand. The other person steps back into *sanchin dachi* with the left leg and blocks the punch with a right *jodan uke* (Figure B). The attack continues by stepping forward again into *sanchin dachi* and punching with the left hand, *chudan zuki* (mid-level punch), at which point the person blocking, having stepped back with his right leg to match the timing of his partner, again into *sanchin dachi*, blocks *chudan uke* (mid-level block) with his left arm (Figure C). With the third punch, step forward and drop into *shiko dachi*; then throw a right *gedan zuki* (low-level punch). The person blocking moves back, also into *shiko dachi,* and blocks the punch with a right *gedan barai* (low-level sweeping block, Figure D). From here the roles are reversed and the practice moves back in the opposite direction.

Some important points to remember are first, the primary purpose of this training is to condition the body to contact. If a block fails, a little impact from the punch should be felt and while great care should be taken when punching to the head, the body blows should carry a little and eventually a fair amount of weight. Secondly, when blocking you should not try to evade the punches but instead blend with the other person's movement with good timing; try to sweep the other person's punch away. Therefore, the backward step should not be thought of as a retreat, but a way of maintaining an appropriate (counter-punching) distance. The people blocking should never move first or out of their own punching range. In the beginning, maintain a strict rhythm of step first, then technique. Later on, if both partners agree, it is possible to go faster and challenge each other at speeds closer to those found in real fighting. If done over the span of say ten or more minutes, *sandan uke barai* taxes the resources of even the fittest and strongest *karateka*.

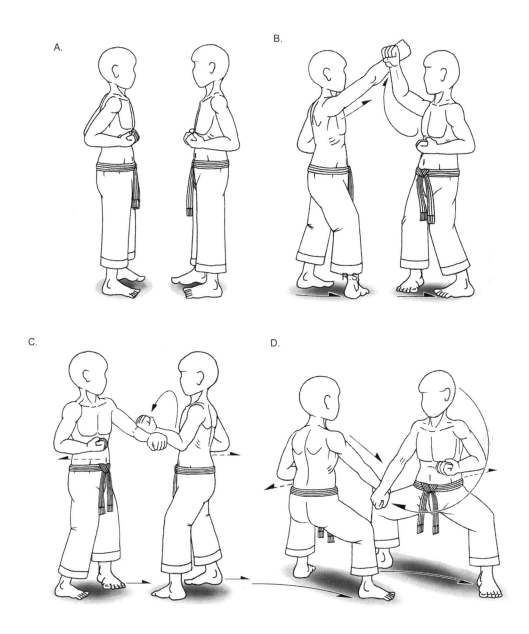

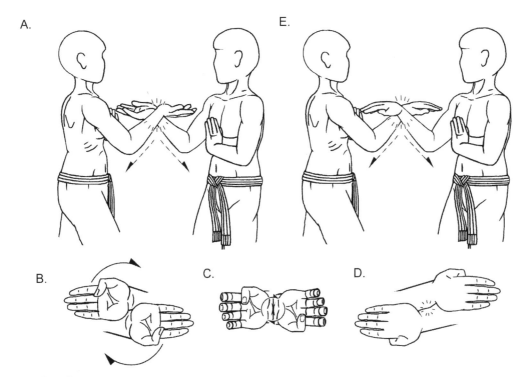

A.

E.

B.

C.

D.

Wrist Rotation

This exercise is done to help gain an understanding of connection *(muchimi)* with the other person and to improve your own ability to anchor yourself to the ground by adopting a low center of gravity. It is a simple-looking exercise that if done properly improves your overall upper body strength and that all-important sense of connection with the ground and with your opponent.

Begin by facing a training partner. Both stand in *migi sanchin dachi* (right leg forward in *sanchin* stance) and place the right wrists together as shown (Figure A). From here, both begin to twist the hands back toward them (Figure B), keeping the palms facing upward until the fingers are pointing directly back toward the face (Figure C). At that point, while continuing to twist, the hands turn over so that the palms are now facing down (Figure D). Each then tries to close down his armpit and in so doing gives the other a slight pull (Figure E). The exercise is repeated in reverse, remembering to keep the wrists together at all times and to keep the hand rotating back toward you each time.

6 AUXILIARY EXERCISES

Hojo Undo Exercises Without Tools

These exercises are not usually done during the course of a regular training session, although of course they could be. If the lifting and impact tools prove difficult to obtain at first, it is possible to begin strengthening the body by spending time doing the following drills. As always, however, caution and common sense need to be exercised when lifting your training partner. Although not as stressful to deal with as the tools, these exercises do offer resistance and help build strength and stamina, timing, and coordination. *Hojo undo* is a training method best suited to people older than sixteen years of age, and while the human body and mind still have some way to go at that age before reaching maturity, with vigilance and careful practice a young adult may find benefit from engaging in a limited form of *hojo undo* training; if this is the case, then some of these exercises are perhaps the best way to start.

What follows are twelve of the exercises we work on during the twice-yearly *gasshuku* at my *dojo*. The list should not be thought of as the only alternatives to working without the tools. They represent no more than a sample of the many exercises we do to prepare the body for the long hours of *karate* training ahead. They can be fun to do, too, of course, although you should never let levity creep too far into training, because dropping your guard in regard to safety provides fertile ground for accidents and injuries. Training partners should ideally be of similar build and weight, and because of the close nature of

The word *gasshuku* means to live or lodge together for a time. In Japanese martial arts, *gasshuku* are, or were, a normal part of the training calendar, and could last as short as a weekend, or as long as two weeks. The purpose of *gasshuku* is to bring students out of their regular life for awhile to concentrate solely on their training. Also, the shared experience of so much training over a relatively short period of time, of eating, cleaning, and sleeping, and of having to exercise patience and show consideration to others is a very important life lesson that many find to be the most difficult part of attending a *gasshuku*. Although not strictly part of Okinawan *karate* tradition, I hold two *gasshuku* each year, one in April and another in October. They mark the month of Chojun Miyagi's birth (April 25, 1888) and the month of his death (October 10, 1953), and they allow me to offer my gratitude and show my appreciation to him for the efforts he made during his lifetime. Without his endeavors, my own life would have been totally different.

some of the drills, training partners should always be of the same gender unless otherwise agreed upon by the female. No figures are given here for the number of times each exercise should be done. The amount of repetitions depends on the fitness level of those doing the training. Too many can lead to injury, and too few to a waste of effort and nothing to show for it. As with all martial arts training, we should work to a level that provides a challenge and then learn to push our own private limits back a little further each day. To do otherwise serves no purpose.

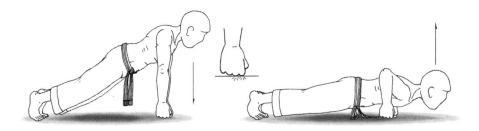

Push-Ups

Begin with a simple push-up, taking care to keep the back straight and the arms close into the sides of the body while it drops in between them. A *karate* push-up should always be done with the fists clenched and with only the index finger and the middle finger of the fist in contact with the floor. This keeps the hand and the arm aligned correctly and safely, and avoids bending or buckling of the wrist joint; it also begins to focus a new student's attention to the impact area of the fist (the first two knuckles) used in a *karate* punch. By keeping the arms in close to the side of the body, with the armpits closed down, the rising and falling approximates the punching action of the arms. Finally, the coordinated breath (inhaling through the nose when you drop and exhaling through the mouth while you push up off the floor) reinforces the pattern of breathing that goes together with the execution of basic techniques.

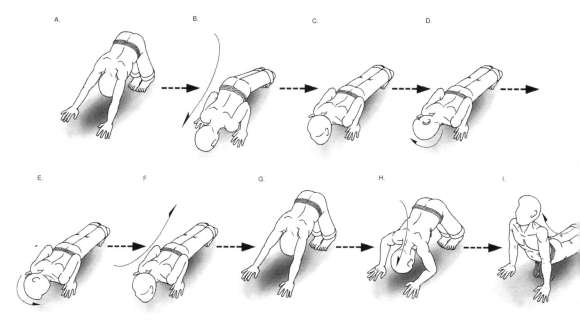

Cat Stretch

This exercise is so called because it reminds people of the way a cat, waking from sleep, often goes through a similar stretching routine with its legs and spine. People who practice yoga will also see distinct similarities in the postures found in this exercise. A cat stretch is divided into two parts, but as you become accustomed to the exercise the link between the two should become invisible as you flow, in harmony with the breath, from one to other.

Begin the first part by placing the balls of the feet and the palms of the hands on the ground in what looks like a really bad push-up position (Figure A). Keep the feet together and stretch the legs and back by gently trying to place the heels on the floor while tucking the head in between the arms and looking up at the *hara*. From here breathe in through the nose and, rocking lightly backward, exhale while scooping the chest to the floor (Figure B) without actually coming into contact with it; straighten out the body, look forward, and end the exhalation and the movement together (Figure C). Turn the head to the right and left in quick succession (Figures D and E), breathing in sharply with each turn, and then look forward (Figure F); breathe out forcibly by squeezing the abdominal muscles (*hara*).

The second part continues from the outward breath that brought the first part to an end. Pushing up and backward with the arms (Figure G) and breathing in as you go, raise the body from the ground and come up on the toes while you roll the body in reverse and scoop back down toward the ground (Figure H). An inward breath accompanies the movement up and away from the floor, and this becomes an outward breath when the body once more moves forward and down. To complete the cat stretch, the back is arched and the head held as if trying to look into the air behind you (Figure I). Hold this posture for a brief moment before gently returning to the starting position. Cat stretches promote rhythmical breathing, controlled body movements, and give a good stretch and strengthening workout to the arms, shoulders, and hamstrings.

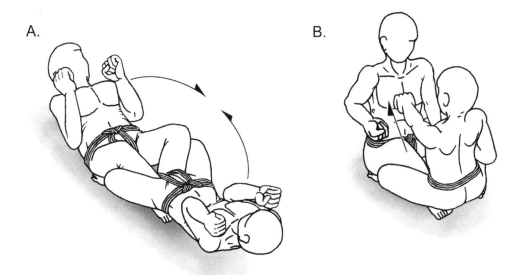

A.

B.

Sit-Up and Punch

Sitting on the floor facing your training partner, both people interlock their legs. This is achieved by the person whose legs are on the inside, turning his feet outward, while the person with his legs on the outside turns his feet inward (Figure A). From this position, both can perform sit-ups. In this version of the exercise, both rise and fall at the same time, and with each sit-up each throws a punch into the body of his training partner (Figure B), both punching with the right arm first and on the next sit-up, with the left. These blows should not be too heavy at first, but later, the intensity of the punch can be increased by mutual agreement.

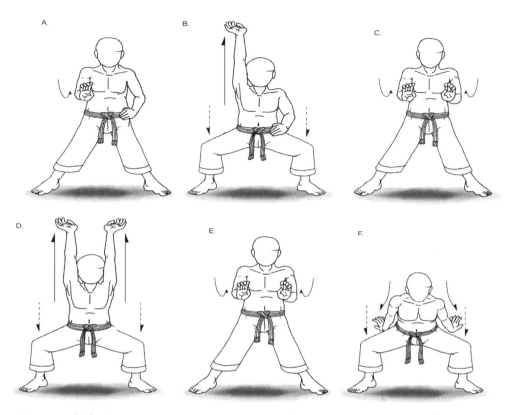

Drop and Thrust

Standing with the legs wide enough apart to drop down into *shiko dachi* (low stance), keep the left hand resting on the thigh and have the right hand open and the arm chambered on the side of the body, as if ready to punch (Figure A). Take a deep breath in through the nose and with a strong exhalation drop the body down into *shiko dachi* and at the same time thrust the right arm directly upward (Figure B). The drop, the thrusting arm, and the outward breath should all conclude at exactly the same time. Hold for just a second before standing back up sharply and chambering the outstretched arm with as much energy as possible, as if striking to the back with an *empi uchi* (elbow strike). This is done with a quick inhalation through the nose. Having completed a number of these exercises, swap hands and repeat the same maneuver with the left hand. Follow this by doing the same again, only this time chambering both arms (Figure C) and thrusting both hands into the air at the same time (Figure D). A fourth version is done by adopting a double arm start position (Figure E), then dropping into *shiko dachi* and striking with a double *shotei uchi* (palm heel strike) to the rear (Figure F).

Resistance Punching

Stand facing your training partner. One person holds out a *chudan zuki* (mid-level punch) with his other arm chambered to the side as normal. The other person holds on to the punching arm, just behind the wrist, and at the same time places his palms resting on the fist of the chambered hand. Taking a deep breath first, the puncher exhales while punching forward; at the same time, his training partner holds on to the retreating arm and pushes against the punch. This is done with sufficient force to make the puncher work hard to overcome the resistance being offered. Once the punch is completed, the person offering the resistance changes his hands over to grip the other wrist and push against the opposite fist of his training partner.

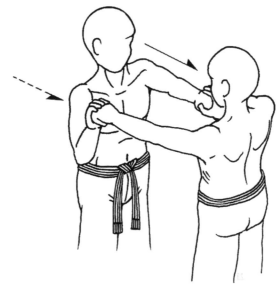

This exercise is done slowly and deliberately for a number of reasons: first, to allow a check to be made of your correct form when punching—wrist and elbow alignment, armpits closed down to connect your body's weight with the technique, harmony of breath and movement, and last but not least, the strong connection with the ground needed to transfer the energy in the punch back into your training partner. If the ground connection is poor, you will find the energy in the punch actually pushed the person punching backward.

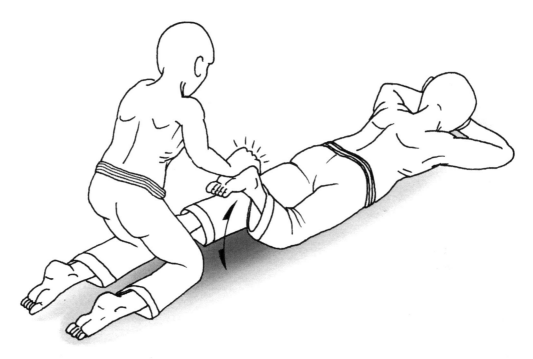

Leg Resistance

One person lies down flat with his chest on the floor and his head resting on the backs of his hands, his legs together and straight. With the training partner holding on to one ankle, the person exercising tries to bend that leg at the knee, bringing the bottom half of the leg to a vertical position against the resistance being presented by the training partner. Once the leg is vertical, the hands move around to offer the same level of resistance when the leg is returned to the floor. From there, change legs and repeat on the other side. Care should be taken not to let the pelvis (hips) leave the floor during the exercise; instead, try to isolate the bottom half of the leg and concentrate on working it against the opposing force.

Similarities to both the *Adho Muka Svanasana* (Downward Facing Dog) and *Bhujangasana* (Cobra) postures of yoga can be found at the start and finish of the cat stretch exercise on page 157, and for me, this is yet one more link pointing to *karate*'s ancient past and the seeds of its distant origin on the Indian sub-continent. The beginning pose in a cat stretch aids the building of shoulder strength and flexibility; it develops a sense of awareness and stretches the spine and the hamstring that runs along the back of the calf muscles in the lower leg. It also rests the heart. The exercise ends in a pose almost exactly like the cobra position, and this too stretches the spine, back, and arms, while opening the chest. It also opens the heart.

Body Catch and Push

Facing each other, one person stands to attention, holding his body stiff with his arms by his side. When ready he falls forward, remaining rigid while he does so. The person catching does so by catching his partner at the shoulders when he drops forward. In the same way as the *kongoken* is used as described in "Kongoken Exercise Four" (page 92), step back while you take the weight of your training partner and then, pushing the hips forward, push him back up to a standing position. Remember to change legs each time you step back to gain a sense of thrusting from both sides of the hip.

In addition, take care not to push too strongly because doing so may result in toppling your training partner backward. It is important to have respect for those we train with and never let our own enthusiasm or lack of *otomo* place others in danger.

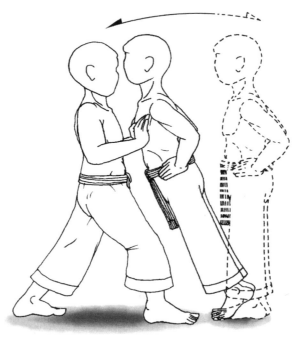

Thrusting the hips is known as *koshi*. The word sounds exactly like the word used for the balls of your foot, but they are not the same. Using the hips without this feeling of *koshi* is a little like pulling a bowstring only halfway back before releasing an arrow.

Otomo means "great friend." On a deeper level, it means developing an ability to be aware of your surroundings, of being in the moment, and to a lesser extent, of anticipation. Here are two examples, the first of bad *otomo*, and the second of good. In the *dojo* the teacher is demonstrating the technique he wants the students to practice; he finishes the demonstration and, within seconds, some students cannot remember what they just saw demonstrated. Outside the *dojo*, a student is walking with his teacher toward a doorway, deep in discussion, and without a word being spoken about the approaching obstacle, the student steps forward and opens the door allowing them both to pass through, the student following his teacher, without breaking the flow of either their walk or conversation.

Heavy Squats

One person stands in *shiko dachi* (low stance) while a training partner, standing behind him, leans his body's weight on his partner's shoulders. From there, the person in *shiko dachi* tries to stand up and drop back down in quick succession. The extra weight from the training partner works the legs and helps build stronger muscles.

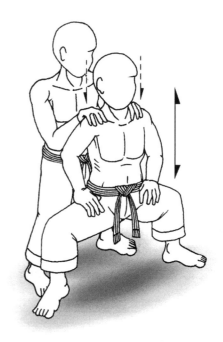

Leg Lift and Push

One person lies on his back on the floor while the other person stands over him. The person on the floor holds onto his training partner's ankles and keeping both legs together and straight swings his feet up toward his partner's stomach, as if to kick him. The person standing catches the ankles and then instantly pushes them back to the ground with some force. The person lying down must not let his feet touch the ground; instead, he immediately swings his legs back up and tries to touch his partner's body. This "contest" works and strengthens the abdominal muscles and helps to coordinate the breathing during quick-fire action. The person doing the leg lift should remember to breathe in when his legs are pushed back to the ground and breathe out when he swings them back up again.

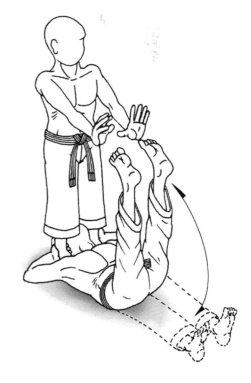

A.   B.

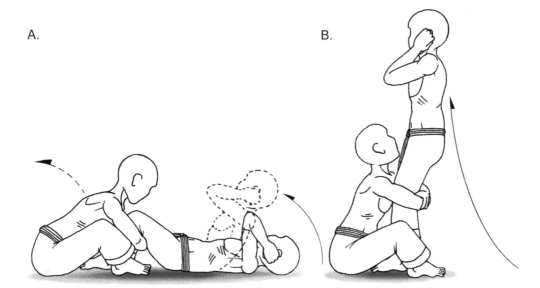

Stand-Ups

With one person lying on his back, knees up, and his feet tucked under his training partner's body, he prepares to do a sit-up. The hands are clenched and held at the side of the face or with fingers clasped behind the head. The other person sits on the ground and places his arms around the back of his partner's knees, anchoring his lower legs to the ground. From this position (Figure A) the person doing the exercise takes in a deep breath before exhaling forcefully while moving into a sit-up. Without stopping, he continues through the sit-up position, focusing on the legs, and stands up (Figure B). At this point the person acting as the anchor should take care not to clash heads while his training partner passes through on the way to standing upright.

Stand to attention for a brief moment before sitting back down and returning to the start position. Great care should be taken when doing this so as not to drop down too heavily on the base of the spine. When ready, take a deep breath—and go again!

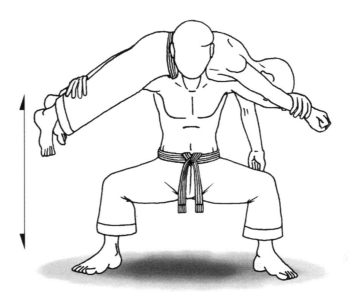

Fireman's Lift and Squat

This exercise is a lot like the heavy squat described earlier; however, it offers much more resistance and requires a greater attention to balance. Because the amount of weight involved is also much greater, this exercise should not be done unless the weight of each training partner is close to equal.

Begin by the person doing the exercise gripping the left wrist of his training partner with his left hand. Lowering his own body by bending the legs, he slips his right arm between the legs of the person being lifted and pulls his partner's left arm over his shoulders and behind his head. This brings the entire weight of your training partner onto your shoulders. Now, standing in *shiko dachi* (low stance) proceed to stand up, and then squat back into *shiko dachi*. Great care should be taken to keep the back as upright as possible to prevent lower back injury. In addition, by adopting a good posture it tests the balance of the person doing the lift.

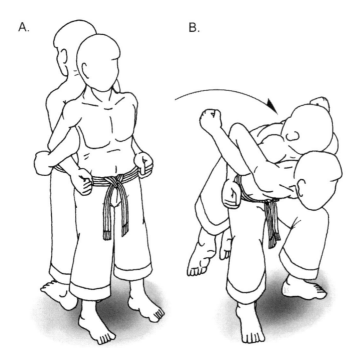

A. B.

Back Lift and Stretch

Standing back to back with your training partner, with the legs in *heiko dachi* (natural stance), interlock your arms (Figure A). From this position one person then bends forward at the waist (Figure B). The person being lifted should relax completely and allow his body's weight to sink. The stretch can be felt across the lower back and should be enjoyed for several seconds before the exercise is reversed. Have consideration for your training partner when changing over and make the transition from one person to the other slowly.

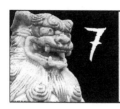

7 OTHER TOOLS AND METHODS

Other Training Tools

As well as the tools discussed in this book, there are more. Actually, the number of variations of each tool that people have and still do come up with makes the inclusion of every tool an impossible task. Nevertheless, I have tried to include all the most commonly used tools, as well as some that have begun to be neglected. The tools in this book are a selection of the equipment I have worked with for over a quarter of a century. There are also some, I think, important tools that deserve a mention here if only because there are, I am sure, individuals still using them and passing on their knowledge to others, and I would not like readers to form the impression that this book is in any way a definitive work on the subject. It is, instead, an introduction to an aspect of traditional *karate* training that I believe is in some danger of being forgotten altogether in the West.

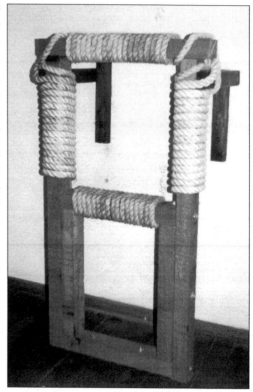

This training device, known as a blocking cube, was used by the author when he lived in Western Australia from 1988 to 1998.

Tetsuwa – Iron Ring

A little over a foot in diameter (30-35 cm), the *tetsuwa* is a descendent of an older ringed tool made from stone and still in use by wrestlers in India today. Some schools of Chinese *Chuan-fa* also use this tool in their normal training routine and there is little doubt, in my mind, that the tool arrived in Okinawa via China.

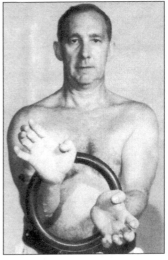

John Porta, a senior teacher of Okinawan *Goju ryu* in America, using the *tetsuwa* to strengthen his arms and wrists.

Ishibukuro – Stone Sack

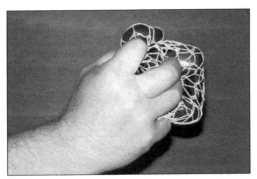

The *ishibukuro* is easy to make, but hard on the fingers.

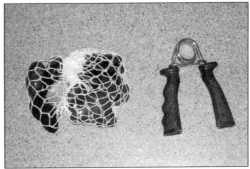

Both of these tools help to increase the gripping power of the hand.

Used to toughen the hands and fingers and improve the grip, the *ishibukuro* is a simple tool to make and use. There are a number of exercises you can do with this tool. Simply by holding it in the hand and then closing the fingers into a tight grip before relaxing again gives a stronger feeling of gripping. Throwing it from one hand to the other (or from one person to another) is also a good way to condition the fingers. I still have one in my *dojo* and use it on a regular basis. I also use the modern equivalent, the sprung handgrip. Each in its own way enhances the strength of the hand and provides me with a challenge.

Small Heavy Bag – Suspended By Rope

Very simple to construct and train with, the small heavy bag is used to condition the body and teach it how to take a blow. Pushing the bag away and allowing it to swing back, impacting on the body, gives the user an opportunity to feel something akin to a real push or punch from an adversary. By changing your stance, angle, and the length of the rope the bag is hanging from, it is possible to target specific parts of the body: the legs, abdomen, or back.

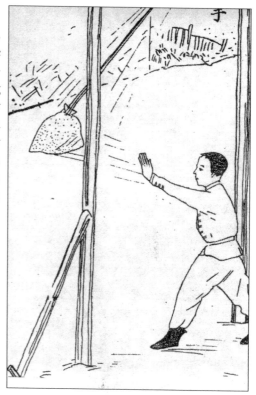

The author uses the same ancient methods seen in this martial text from China.

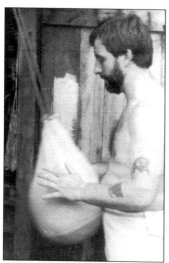

Swinging a bag or ball filled with cement and allowing it to land on various parts of the body, conditions the mind and body to the effects of impact.

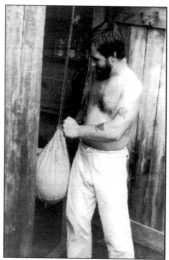

A favorite target for attack, conditioning the legs in this way helps build confidence and an ability to continue on, even when struck.

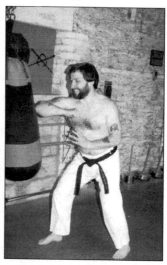

A heavy kick bag is an excellent tool for all *karateka*. It allows movement and requires the user to use his strength efficiently.

Torso Wheel – Roller

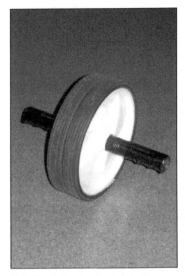

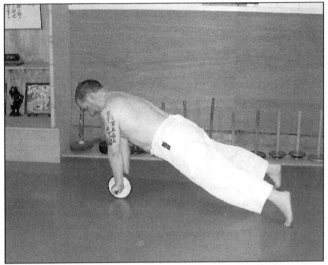

This simple-looking tool works the arms, leg, and torso. It also requires good breath control.

The author still uses this tool for enhancing arm strength and balance, as well as keeping the torso strong.

It might be advisable to purchase one of these from a good sports store although making one should not be beyond the capabilities of those who wish to keep in the spirit of *hojo undo* and make their tools from recycled materials. A wheel with a handle on either side may look simple enough, but this tool proves to be a tough adversary for the abdominal muscles. If you do make this tool yourself, it is advisable to use a length of steel as the handle because wood can and often does break.

Sanchin Bar – Spring Bar

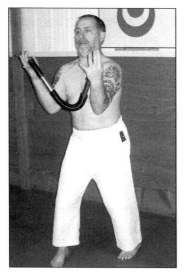

The amount of energy captured in the tool during this exercise means great care must be taken not to let one end slip from the hands.

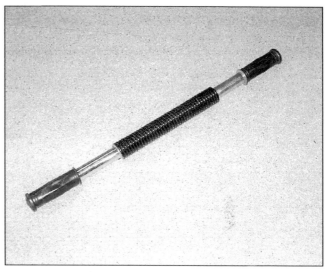

A massive amount of energy is stored in this tool during its use. Great care should be taken when working with it.

Although this tool can be made from an old coiled spring and two lengths of wood or steel for the handles, I think the forces involved are so strong that in most cases it is better to buy a well-constructed tool from a good sports store. Alternatively, you can do what I do and search the swap meets, car boot (trunk) sales, and garage sales because these are often where you can find the best *hojo undo* tools.

Impact Training – Tapping Stick

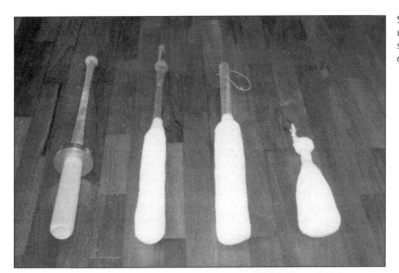

Some of the 'tapping sticks' used by Hokama *sensei*'s students at his Kenshinkan *dojo* in Nishihara, Okinawa.

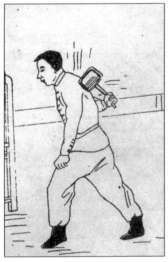

Impact training has long been considered important in Chinese martial arts.

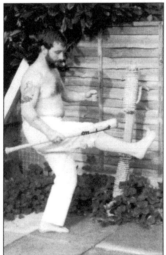

The author using a baseball bat to 'tap' his shin during training at Richard Barrett's *dojo* in Hertfordshire, England, c. 1987.

This training can be done with almost any piece of wood and is just a matter of striking various parts of the body on a regular basis to build up a sense of familiarity. *Karate* cannot be understood without an appreciation of impact upon our own body, and this is a simple and effective way to introduce it. The object of the exercise is to tap, with attitude, but not to hit yourself as hard as possible.

Other Training Methods

Running and Swimming. As well as the tools and exercises shown in this book, there are many other ways to supplement your feeling for *karate*. Your ability to coordinate the breath and the body to run or swim well are directly transferable to *karate*, as is the ability needed to do each of these activities in a controlled and relaxed manner. In doing so, you will discover that harmonious balance between a hard-working body and a quiet, calm mind. Like a graceful swan gliding, seemingly without effort, across the surface of the water, a *karateka*'s technique should appear natural and relaxed, almost effortless in fact. Look below the surface of the water, however, and just as we see the swan's legs are working hard to propel it, intelligent observation of a well-trained *karateka* will also reveal the hidden effort needed to allow the body to move with such apparent ease.

Skipping. This too is an activity that brings the trinity of mind, body, and breath into focus and is something not to be ignored. Like a good many other activities it appears simple: child's play! Nevertheless, it is no accident that professional fighters have used this type of training for as long as they have. Its benefits can be judged by how quickly it peels away the ego and brings us face to face with our true self. Five minutes into a fifteen-minute skip is a place where a *karateka*'s self-image is often tested to a breaking point. For by this time, a mind in disharmony with the body will begin to falter, and the *karateka* comes face to face with the fundamental challenge of training and life itself: to quit or to carry on. At such times it is important to look for a way through and not a way out. The struggle we face when we find ourselves in situations like this and how we resolve that struggle is exactly why the fighting arts have value for us far beyond mere fighting.

Climbing. This activity (with all the inherent safety measures in place) not only enhances the agility and strength of the arms and legs, but of the mind too. Thinking clearly under pressure, remaining calm when facing the fear of falling, and digging deep within yourself to reach the summit are attributes also found in people who have come to understand *karate*. Strenuous physical activity, counter-balanced by a calm mind, is a potent and real weapon in a world where we are being constantly bombarded with images and ideas that point us away from personal commitment. To stand before a difficult climb and to reach the top by your own means is a powerful affirmation of your own ability to deal with life.

Others may well have climbed the same rock face before us, but none will have done it precisely as we did. Others may have come to understand *karate* before us, but none will have reached that understanding exactly as we did. Others may be living life in great contentment, but again, none will be doing so by the same means as we, for our life and our training are, by their very nature, ours alone to experience.

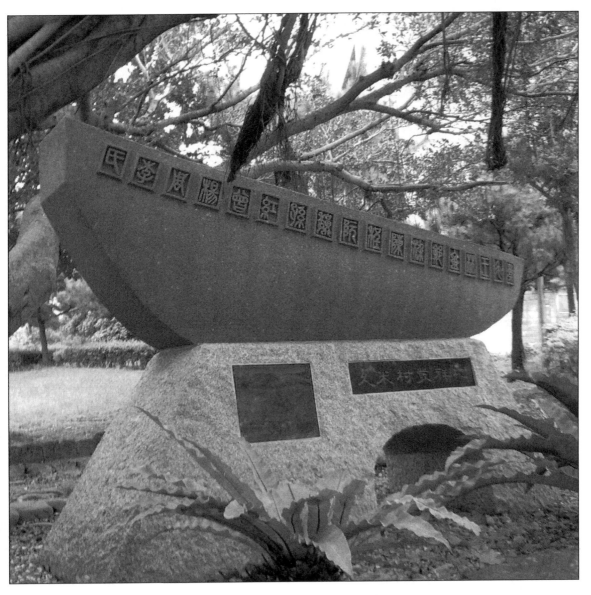

Memorial to China's 36 Families.

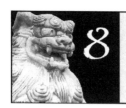

8 COMMENTS ON HOJO UNDO FROM OKINAWAN KARATE MASTERS

Since I began traveling to Okinawa in 1984, I have been privileged to meet many great *karate* teachers over the years. Some have had a worldwide following, while others have not, but the majority of them have had something in common—their sincere love for the fighting arts of their homeland and their willingness to share what they know with others. It is beyond the scope of this book to detail the many conversations I have had with all of them, but I thought I would include a brief extract from just two of these exchanges to provide an incentive to others to seek out such teachers and perhaps have their own conversations.

Tetsuhiro Hokama sensei, 10ᵗʰ Dan, Goju ryu

Michael Clarke (MC): *How important is hojo undo training in karate?*

Tetsuhiro Hokama (TH): Well, as you know, in older times masters such as Kanryo Higaonna *sensei*, and Chojun Miyagi *sensei* went to China, and there they were training very hard every day. This was the Fuken style of fighting which became our *Goju ryu karate* when these people came back to Okinawa. While in China, they found out about *hojo undo* and so this became a very important part of training. Today, some people think that *karate* is just like any other sport, baseball, basketball, etc., but *hojo undo* is very spe-

cial and so this makes *karate* very different from sport. The way we breathe in and out using these tools, for example, maybe in the sport kind of *karate hojo undo* is not so important, but for *budo karate* it is very important. Of course, all sports people want to know "how" their body works. So this is the same, but in *Goju ryu* we try to stay soft in our body as we breathe in, and become strong when we breathe out, for example in *sanchin kata*.

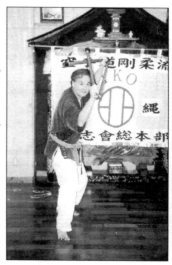

Tetsuhiro Hokama using a three section staff.

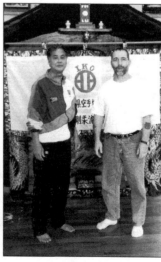

The author with Tetsuhiro Hokama at the Kenshinkan *dojo*.

We have *kata* in *Goju ryu,* but if you don't train *hojo undo* too the *kata* is no good; it looks (feels) very bad! We have *sanchin* and *tensho kata* too. These are like the foundation of a house that is maybe five levels high. The foundation is *sanchin kata*, and *hojo undo* is the foundation support. Above that we have the *kata* to form the different levels of the house. *Kumite* forms the roof, and the outside walls are formed by the *kata* application. This is how we build a *karate* house! But, most importantly, we must have strong foundations. This idea of training in *Goju ryu* is Chojun Miyagi *sensei's* idea.

In 1392, thirty-six families from China came to Okinawa and settled in the Kume area. They brought with them the practice of *kenpo* and also the *Bubishi* (a book much revered by Okinawan *karateka*). They had many fighting techniques and training methods that were secret. Mr. Miyagi's teacher was Kanryo Higaonna, his teacher before going to China as a teenager was Seisho Arakaki, his teacher was master Yabu, and his teacher was Master Hokama. This is the earliest time I can find my family name recorded. I don't think we are related however. But before Hokama *sensei*, his teacher was a Chinese descendent from the thirty-six families.

MC: *Can children train hojo undo?*

TH: Yes it is okay, but you have to be careful what they do. Their bodies are still soft and forming so you cannot train like adults do, but they can do their kicking and punching against a soft pad. For them *hojo undo* involves stretching, jumping, skipping, and things like that. They practice *sanchin kata*, but again, their training is not like an adult's. But *sanchin* is the *Goju ryu* foundation, so they must learn the style.

Kosuke Yonamine sensei, 9th Dan, Shohei ryu Karatedo

MC: *Yonamine sensei, can you please talk about your training in hojo undo?*

Kosuke Yonamine (KY): Yes, well, I always liked to do this kind of training. We used wood to condition the different parts of the body, like the arms, legs, shins, toes, etc. We hit these parts of the body many times. Now, of course, I am older so I don't do as much as I once did, but I still train this way. I think it is important to condition your body, not only so you can do *karate*, but you see, because we are not all born with the same bodies. Some people are naturally big and strong, but some of us are not.

As I started to get better at *karate* I felt I had to get stronger. So, step-by-step, I increased the conditioning to make myself as strong as I could be. It is important not only to be fit, but to be strong also. If you get hit during training, or in real life, you should

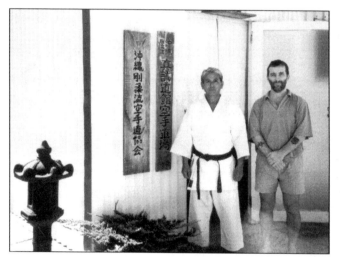
Kosuke Yonamine and author at the Shinseidokan dojo Australia.

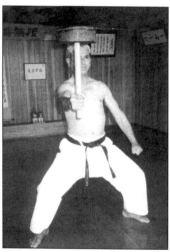
Kosuke Yonamine at the author's Shinseidokan dojo.

be strong enough to take a bit of this so that you can continue. It is no good if you stop because you have been hit. I was taught from the beginning that the human body has some points that are weak, and so I should try to hit these points. There are many such places on the body—all over! When I train in *kata* I always feel I am hitting these areas; this is important. This is also why some conditioning is necessary for fingers and toes.

MC: *What kind of special training did you do for your fingers and toes?*

KY: For my toes, I kicked concrete and wood, and I also kicked the *makiwara* and sandbags too. Sometimes these were soft sandbags and *makiwara* with a lot of "give" in them, but these always led to kicking more solid sandbags and stronger *makiwara*. As well as these things, I have always used the hard floor to push against with my toes. Many hours spent doing these things have over time given me a stronger body, and certain parts of my body are now very strong. Because I trained properly and did not do stupid things with my body, I still have good health and suffer no ill effects from this kind of training. I have no problems with my hands or my feet, and they are still very strong.

A Last Word

This book, if it works as it was intended, will shine a light back onto an aspect of traditional *karate* training that has slowly slipped from view due to the overwhelming glare of sporting and commercial interests. *Hojo undo* is not *karate* style or martial art specific; Okinawan *karateka* have always supplemented the training they did inside the *dojo* with various activities outside of it, as did their *kobudo* cousins. Stories of people performing their *kata* in the strong winds that hit the island each year or training while standing waist deep in the ocean, and running up and down the many hills and along the beaches of their island home bear testimony to this training and form part of the rich oral history of *karate* and *kobudo* on the island. Today this kind of *hojo undo* continues much as it has always done. Although the vast majority of people training in Okinawan fighting arts around the world these days are not in fact Okinawan, I believe it is important to maintain a similar attitude toward our training (taking into account the differences in the respective societies) as our Okinawan counterparts if we are to maintain a connection to their culture, and through that, to traditional *karate* and *kobudo* and the masters of old. To understand the new is to understand the old, as the Okinawans might say. This is, I believe, the conduit by which the "tradition" that traditional *budoka* speak of is passed from one generation to the next, and it is for this reason that this book has been written: to encourage those who may be interested in the traditional Okinawan methods of training to look beyond the confines of the fighting techniques found in any particular style or association and embrace the concept of *hojo undo* in all its many forms.

The practice of traditional *hojo undo* is not just a handy "body-building" adjunct to the fighting techniques of a particular martial art; it runs much deeper than that. The tools, properly made and with sufficient weight, will test the user to his limits and provide opportunities to grow and mature: hallmarks of a truly traditional martial artist. The trinity of *shin gi tai* (mind, body, spirit), and the harmony with which they function within us, is a concept fundamental to the understanding of all Japanese and Okinawan *budo*, and is clearly apparent in the practice of *hojo undo*. You cannot manipulate a tool effectively without employing it. This book, although not conclusive in its coverage of every type of tool to be found in the *dojo*s of Okinawa, has been written with the aim of pointing readers in the right direction in the hope that they may discover for themselves the wealth of understanding that flows from such training. Understanding, not only of their body and how it works, but also of the blending of the breath, the body, and the mind (intention), and the enormous energy such a combination has to offer, *hojo undo* gives us an insight into something Okinawan martial artists have known and understood for generations and allows everyone who trains this way to make yet another small step forward in their own pursuit of *budo* and understanding of the "self."

Endnotes

Chapter 1: Introduction

1. According to the account given by Dr. Clive Layton in his book *Shotokan Dawn*, vol. 1 (Llangefni, Wales: Mona Books, 2007), p. 36, Henri D. Plée began his martial arts training in *judo* shortly after the Second World War and became the sixteenth person in France to be awarded *shodan* in that art. An article in the October 1948 edition of *Life* magazine inspired his interest in *karate*. The article and accompanying photographs showing two students from Wasada University, Gojuro Harada and Hiroshi Kamata, sparring captured his imagination. In the winter of 1953, Plée met Donn Draeger, a former major in the United States Marine Corps who would in later years become famous throughout the world for his writings on the martial arts. Draeger was able to help Plée acquire a copy of a short film (15 min., 42 sec.) showing Masayoshi Nakayama training with Isao Obata. The following year, 1955, Plée (who was clearly not shy about his grasp on all things martial) wrote his first book on *karate* and called it *Vaincre ou mourir l'esprit et la technique du: Karate-Do* published in Paris (cited on page 36 of Dr. Clive Layton's book, *Shotokan Dawn*). In 1955, Plée became a founding member of the Federation Francaise de Karate et Boxe Libre, becoming its first secretary general.

   In his book, *Karate: Beginner to Black Belt,* (London: Foulsham, 1967), a photo of the youthful looking Frenchman appears alongside a list of his accomplishments and reads as follows: 5th *Dan Karate*, 4th *Dan Judo*, 2nd *Dan Aikido*, Honorary President of the French Federation of Judo and Associated Disciplines, and President of the Karate Technical Commission.

2. Masao Kawasoe was born to Japanese parents in occupied Korea on June 13, 1945. He entered Takushoku University, Tokyo, and joined the *karate* club where, upon graduation, he joined the Japan Karate Association and completed its instructor's training course. His first professional post was to the island of Taiwan, his second to Madagascar, and finally to Great Britain in 1974, where he has lived ever since.

3. Throughout his biography, written by Dr. Clive Layton (*Masao Kawasoe, 8th Dan,* Llangefni, Wales: Mona Books, 2008), Kawasoe describes some of his encounters with training equipment. On page 36 he talks about his time training with Tsuyama *sensei*, before he entered university:

   I wanted a mae geri (front kick) like my teacher's and so I would do the exercises at home as well, every day, at least one hundred lifts each leg with the heavy iron geta. I used to practice kicks on the sandbag that hung in the dojo too. I did a lot of bag work…. I sometimes punched with weights, keeping the weights underside, building muscle, and I experimented generally, though I never sought to strengthen my nukite (spear hand) by driving my fingertips into sand, or anything like that. I also built a makiwara in the garden and would face it every day with punches, gyaku zuki (reverse hip straight punch) mainly. Makiwara training helps to forge the fist (seiken)…. the punching pad was made of straw. When I found the makiwara, my experimentation with other training aids largely faded because the makiwara has everything the karateka needs really, at least for punches and strikes.

   With the exception of the *makiwara*, by the time he became a student at Takushoku University his training involved hardly any *hojo undo* at all. On page 73, he goes on to say:

   Inside Takushoku dojo there was a sand bag used for kicking and a mirror for checking form. There was a good relationship between the judo and karate members and we'd sometimes go to their dojo and practice with weights. We didn't use chiishi, that's Okinawan, Goju ryu, but we did use a special heavy club (as seen in Nakayama's book), a bit like a large baseball bat, that we'd bring down over our heads and stop, suddenly, like the bokken that kendoka use. I found this very good practice for focus, both shime and kime.

4. George E. Mattson is a legendary figure in Western *karate*. He trained under Kanei Uechi, son of the founder of *Uechi ryu*, in the mid-1950s while stationed in Okinawa with the American military. In his second book *Uechi Ryu Karate-do: Classical Chinese Okinawan Self-Defense,* (Newton, MA: Peabody Publishing, 1974), he states that he wrote his first book in 1958. If this is the case, I'm left wondering why it took a further five years to see it published. Be that as it may, when *The Way of Karate* first hit the bookshops in 1963 (I have a first edition hardback copy), it must have appeared strange and esoteric. It has to be said that at the time of writing, Mattson's skill in *karate* was somewhat limited, and this is borne

out in many of the photographs throughout the book. Nevertheless, what captures my attention is not the lack of athletic ability seen in some of the images, but the extraordinary effort to which Mattson went to present *karate* to a Western public with as little hype and show as possible. In fact, a large portion of the text deals with subjects other than the fighting techniques. Chapters discussing such topics as "What is *Karate*?" and "What *Karate* is Not," and "*Karate* and *Zen*" would still find value in the reading material of *karateka* today. To my mind, it is truly amazing that a Western student of *karate* was able to write such a book as this, some fifty years ago. Perhaps he received assistance from Anthony Mirakian *sensei*, who had been stationed on Okinawa for six years during the 1950s, which allowed him to gain so much insight. Who knows? Certainly, Mirakian has vivid memories of helping Mattson with the book and related as much in a telephone conversation I had with him in September 2008. Regardless of who helped whom, the competitive element was on the rise. Little more than a decade after this book was published, Bruce Lee would explode upon the screen and, with the help of motion picture fantasy and television, change the face of Oriental martial arts forever.

5. Kanryo Higaonna (pronounced Higashionna in the Okinawan dialect *hogen*) was born in Nishimura village, not far from the capital of Okinawa, on March 10, 1853. The son of a merchant trader whose father, Kanyo, sailed to and fro around the smaller islands off the Okinawan coast buying and selling firewood, the young Higaonna grew strong from the work he had to do while helping his father make a living, and by all accounts the two had an exceptionally close bond. Tragically, while Kanryo was still a young man, his father died suddenly.* Sometime after that, around 1875, Kanryo left Okinawa for China where like many of his fellow countrymen, he settled in the city of Fuzhou. Various historians have reported that he remained in China for as little as eight years and for as long as fifteen, although new research seems to indicate that he may actually have been abroad for as little as three years.†

---

* According to a story told to me many years ago by Morio Higaonna (no relation), Kanryo's father was killed in a knife fight. Discovering who had killed his father, the 14-year-old Kanryo vowed to take revenge when he was older and later took off for China to learn the skills necessary to fulfill that commitment. Upon his return, however, he learned that the man had died only a few days earlier. The intervening years of hard training had mellowed Kanryo's character and he no longer held a desire to kill anyone. Learning of the miserable plight of the man's widow and children, he attended the funeral and made an offering of condolence money in accordance with Okinawan custom.

I have come across this same story from other sources where the name of the person involved was not divulged. So the veracity of the above tale must be treated with some caution. Okinawa has a long and well-established history of legends and apocryphal accounts emanating from its martial traditions that may or may not have happened in quite the same way as the story tells it. Personally, I enjoy listening to these stories; however, such tales must be taken with a very large pinch of salt. Real research in order to grasp a clear understanding of past, people, and events takes much time and effort and is unfortunately beyond the reach of many who have limited resources. Thankfully, there are people we can look to, who have the capacity and the competence to unearth and sort out the facts from the fables.

† Information regarding Kanryo Higaonna's stay in China and the kind of martial art he taught upon his return to Okinawa are explored in the article, "The Myths and Facts Surrounding Higashionna Kanryo," by Mario McKenna *Dragon Times Magazine* 19 (2000). Further light is shed on this question on his Internet blog in July 2008, when McKenna's translation of Iken Tokashiki's research into the life of Kanryo Higaonna is presented as an extract from the 1987 yearbook of the Gohakukai, a karate organization founded by Tokashiki. On page 122 of the yearbook, Tokashiki wrote:

> [T]he grandson of Kanryo Higaonna stated that "My grandfather was against the Ryukyu Kingdom becoming part of mainland Japan. He travelled to Fuzhou with others to petition the Ching government requesting assistance and support for the Ryukyu Kingdom. He stayed in China for three years where he worked as a bamboo craftsman and at the same time studied toudi (old Okinawan name for karate). My father-in-law told me this story."

To confirm the story, Gohakukai members met Urasoe city library curator, Dr, Kurayoshi, and Mr. Tana from the Naha City Cultural Promotion Division. They wanted to hear their expert opinions on the historical background of the era. The two men stated that during the 1870s around the time Kanryo Higaonna was known to have gone to China, travel to Fuzhou to study was restricted, and that going to China to study *toudi* (*karate*) was not permitted. Still, many people did travel to their giant neighbor to lobby for support against Okinawa being annexed by Japan. According to the expert opinions of Mr. Tana and Dr. Kurayoshi, it was under these circumstances that Kanryo Higaonna managed to leave Okinawa and travel to Fuzhou. This explanation of events creates a counterpoint to the suggestion that Kanryo Higaonna studied martial arts in China for ten or fifteen years, as some well-known Okinawan writers have suggested.

Regardless of how long he was away from his homeland, all agree that during his stay in China he studied the martial arts for four or five hours almost every day. When he was not training, it was only to work, sleep, eat, and complete the cleaning and household chores set him by his teacher, Ryu Ryu Ko (also known as Xie Zhong Xian, 1852-1930). If the dates to be found are accurate, his new Chinese teacher was only one year older than he, and Kanryo had already been training since his teenage years in the martial arts of his countrymen under the tutelage of Seisho Arakaki of Kume village. Yet it is widely accepted by *karate* historians that the training he received in China elevated him to a different level in skill and understanding.

Returning to Okinawa sometime in the later years of the 1870s, he was no longer the same young man who had left his home but a man that was, even then, considered one of the most skilled empty-hand fighters on the island. Such was his kicking ability alone that some people gave him the nickname *Ashi-no-Higaonna* (legs Higaonna). He was later bestowed with other names too: *Tanmai* (a term of respect and affection), *Bushi* (Gentleman Warrior), and *Kensei* (Fist Saint), being three of them. Keeping a low profile for many years after his return home and keeping his abilities to himself, it took countless approaches by local officials and ordinary citizens alike to persuade him to begin passing on what he had learned in China.

Chapter 2: Preparation Exercises

6. An excellent example of this being executed by Hirokazu Kanazawa *sensei* can be seen on page 246 (photo 27-B) of his book *Shotokan Karate International Kata*,1982.

Chapter 3: Lifting Tools

7. Tetsuhiro Hokama *sensei*, 10th *Dan Goju ryu karatedo*, is head of the Okinawa *Goju ryu Kenshin kai*, and also the owner of Okinawa's only *karate* museum. Located in Nishihara, close to the University of the Ryukyus, it is open by appointment only, and visitors must first telephone ahead to arrange a visit. Hokama *sensei* is a warm and enthusiastic guide, speaks very good English, and often acts as the historical adviser for documentary filmmakers and mainland TV crews who visit Okinawa. The small donation of two hundred Yen he asks to view the collection is rewarded by the staggering amount of artifacts and photographs on display. A prolific writer with numerous books and magazine articles to his credit, he has produced several instructional DVDs and appeared in a number of documentaries. As well, he is a master calligrapher of the Shungan School; his skills in the art of *Shodo* (the way of writing with the brush) are known and appreciated around the world.

8. Along with the large *jori* (heavy wooden clubs) used by Indian wrestlers to build powerful shoulders and gripping strength, they also train with the *gada* (mace), a heavy stone ball fixed to the end of a length of wood measuring about a meter (thirty-nine inches) or more in length; the *gar nal* (stone wheel), a doughnut-shaped ring of stone the size of a car tire; the *sumtola*, a heavy log with handles cut into it; and the *mallakhamb* (wrestlers pole), a post set into the ground reaching over three meters (ten feet) into the air, and upon which the wrestlers swing, climb, and twist their bodies and limbs. The senior wrestlers also train with a set of *nail jori*, a large pair of clubs studded with nails. One touch to the body from these during the spinning and turning exercises and the nails will cut deeply into the wrestlers' flesh.

9. He is known in Japan as Daruma. In his book, *Traditional Karate*, 1985, Morio Higaonna writes that when the Indian monk Bodhidharma took up residence at the *Shaolin-szu* (Shaolin monastery) in the Song-shan Mountains of Honan Province around the year A.D. 520, he found the Chinese monks there too unfit to endure the long hours of meditation, and so he devised a number of exercises designed to make them more healthy in both mind and body. These, it is supposed, formed the genesis of *Shaolin* boxing, a method of fighting now known the world over. According to Higaonna, Bodhidharma produced two texts at this time, *Yi Jing Jin* (Japanese: *Ekkinkyo*) and *Xi Shui Jin* (Japanese: *Senzuikyo*), consisting of eighteen *kata* (exercises) and two *sutras*. In the *Yi Jing Jin*, instructions on how to do a number of physical exercises and special breathing methods that would increase the monks' physical strength were given. The second text focused more on the mental and spiritual strength of the monks. Although seemingly concerned with two totally different aspects of the human condition, together these texts pointed to the same goal: a healthy body enhancing a healthy mind. This harmony was going to be necessary if the monks were ever to gain enlightenment.

10. The weaving of fabric by the women of Okinawa is a well-established tradition stretching back centuries. Various styles of weaving became established, and distinct designs emerged that can still be found today. As well as the weaving of cloth, a particular dying process also emerged. Known as *Bingata*, its use of

primary colors saw this process originally reserved for clothes worn by the royal household. However, it is now a much-loved part of Okinawan traditional life and its use can be found all over the island. *Shuri ori* style weaving developed due to influences from the surrounding Southeast Asian countries with which the Ryukyu Kingdom traded. Other styles to develop include *Kasuri, Hana ori* and *Hanakura ori.*

11. In the nineteenth-century Okinawa, there were, in fact, no *karate dojo* as we would know them today. Instead, training was conducted late at night or in the early hours of the morning, in hidden groves and other out-of-the-way places. Graveyards seem to have been a favorite place for this activity, and this may have had something to do with wanting to keep things secret. After all, you were not likely to have the training interrupted by a casual observer if you were surrounded by graves at 2:00 A.M. As Okinawa became ever more absorbed into the nation of Japan and with the advance of Japanese culture throughout the Ryukyu Kingdom, its *dojo*-based martial arts instructional template began to impose itself on the in-digenous martial arts. *Karate* began to emerge from the shadows in the last years of the 1800s, and *karate dojo* began to appear in neighborhoods all over the island.

12. Although a number of schools of Okinawan *karate* share similar names for some of their *kata*, the actual *kata* itself can be quite dissimilar, hence the notification of these *kata* being the *Goju ryu* version. For example, the *sanchin, sanseiru* and *seisan kata* of *Goju ryu* and *Uechi ryu* are very different. In this case the reason for the same name being attributed to training patterns that clearly look and feel different may stem from the fact that both Kanryo Higaonna, 1853-1915, and Kanbun Uechi, 1877-1948 (the teacher of *Goju ryu*'s founder Chojun Miyagi, and the founder of *Uechi ryu karate* respectively), trained for an extended period of time in Southern China. Although they studied under different *sifu* (teachers), Higaonna with Xie Zhong Xian* (also known as Ryu Ryu Ko) and Uechi with Chou Tsu Ho (also known as Shushiwa), they are thought to have studied similar methods of *Chuan-fa* (Chinese boxing).

13. Chojun Miyagi arrived in Honolulu, Hawaii, on May 3, 1934, having sailed there from Tokyo onboard the steamship, *Tatsuta Maru*, and stayed in the islands until returning home in February of the following year. Invited there by Chinyei Kinjo, head of a local Japanese language newspaper and a fellow Okinawan, he celebrated his 46th birthday while on the voyage and upon his arrival toured the islands giving lectures, demonstrations, and even teaching a small number of people, sometimes in their homes. This was not a money-making venture for Miyagi *sensei*; it was more of a cultural goodwill tour aimed at boosting the morale of the many Okinawan families who had immigrated to the islands since the beginning of the twentieth century.

14. Whether or not Chojun Miyagi actually brought a *kongoken* home with him from Hawaii, or just returned with the idea in his head, is unclear. However, by the time the photograph on the opposite page was taken in the year Showa 17 (the photograph was taken on December 21, 1942, and shows Miyagi *sensei* with students from the Naha Commercial High School), the *kongoken* was clearly in use. The student second from the right in the back row can be seen holding one. It is edge on to the camera and partly hidden by the student's own body, but it is clearly a *kongoken*. Also in the photograph are a *tan, chiishi, ishisashi, nigiri gami,* several barbells, a *tou,* and a portable *makiwara*.

15. Charles C. Goodin is a *karateka* based in Honolulu, Hawaii. A world-renowned writer and researcher of *karate* on the islands, he also operates the Hawaii Karate Museum, a repository of great stature and interest to all serious researchers regarding *karate*'s history. In 1997 he established the Hikiri *dojo* where he teaches *Shorin ryu karatedo* and *Yamani ryu bojutsu*.

Chapter 4: Impact Tools

16. On page 24 of the October 2008 issue of *Shotokan Karate Magazine*, Kousaku Yokata, a 6th *Dan* student of *Shotokan karate* had this to say about *Shotokan karate* myths:

> *We know that the makiwara came from Okinawa but we have little documentation to support its history. I discovered, to my surprise, that this tradition is only a hundred years old since its invention. It is believed that Matsumura Sokon (1809–1899) initially invented the makiwara and Itosu Anko (Master Funakoshi's sensei, 1830–1915) popularized it in the early 1900s. Matsumura sensei*

---

* Patrick McCarthy made this important discovery some years ago and his findings, along with an actual photograph of Xie Zhong Xian himself, were published in *Fighting Arts International Magazine* 87 (1994): 47. Before this time even senior *Goju ryu karate figures* in Okinawa had no idea of Ryu Ryu Ko's real name, let alone what he looked like.

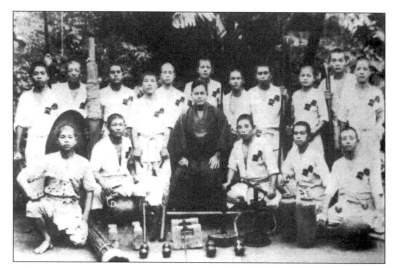

This photograph, taken in 1942, shows the *kongoken* was being used by Chojun Miyagi's students after his return from Hawaii. The student standing second from the right (back row) is holding one.

trained in kenjutsu called Jigen ryu of Satsuma. Jigen ryu is a unique style and its main practice is to hit a wooden bar that is held horizontally with a bokken (wooden sword). Historians believe that Matsumura got the idea of the makiwara from Jigen-ryu practice.

In his attempt to show that the *makiwara* is a fairly recent addition to *karate's* traditional training methods, Yokata makes the case that the tool is not only unnecessary to the acquisition of fighting skills, but can in fact be counterproductive. He qualifies his position by stating that, "We (*yudansha* – black belt students) do not have to have calluses on our fists to knock someone down." He goes on to say, "We must truly understand one important fact here. The characteristics of the human body are totally different from those of wooden posts (*makiwara*) and punching bags." He concludes this part of the article with the thought, "We must wonder why most martial artist don't pick up the *makiwara*."

There is a short answer to his last observation, and that is, training on the *makiwara* is often very painful. The longer and perhaps less cynical explanation has more to do with people misunderstanding the role this particular tool plays in the overall conditioning and education of a *karateka*. The *makiwara* was never intended to approximate a human being. Nor was it designed to propagate the large knuckles, mentioned by Yokata, that often appear as a result of frequent contact by the first two knuckles of the fist slamming into the target area. That he should use such arguments to support his claim that the *makiwara* is unnecessary misses the point entirely.

Like the other tools found in the practice of *hojo undo,* the *makiwara* plays a particular and important role in the conditioning of the mind, as well as bringing focus to bear on certain physical attributes needed to deliver a decisive blow. For reasons best known to them, the early Japanese *karateka* took to hitting the *makiwara* with as much enthusiasm as they displayed in their abandonment of the other tools. And just as they changed the emphasis of *karate* training away from the in-depth study of *kata* and onto the practice of endless basic techniques, they also managed to shift the focus of *makiwara* training away from its original purpose, and turned it into some kind of testosterone fueled display of "guts."

Regardless of when the *makiwara* was 'invented' its value to the *karateka* of Okinawa is beyond doubt. Its use has helped them to develop powerful punches that belie their diminutive stature and, along with the other tools found in *hojo undo,* it has helped shape the character of those who would face it.

17. On page 82 of his autobiography, *Karate, My Life*, the legendary Kanazawa *sensei* recalls his early encounters with the *makiwara* as follows;

> *The most basic form of training is makiwara tsuki (punching a makiwara or hitting board). This exercise conditions fingers and knuckles, and also helps develop abdominal strength. Legs, hips and lower back are strengthened and you develop finely tuned, supple muscles. Back then we made our own makiwara. There was a rice merchant near the University where I would go and get*

some empty straw rice bags and use them as the main material. The merchant always looked puzzled as to what we could possibly want the empty bags for. Once we made the makiwara covered with straw, we would attach it to the post in the ground and reinforce it. All done.

Nowadays makiwara tsuki is practiced quite scientifically with emphasis placed on speed and correct use of strength. In those days, however, we did not think so much about the finer details and just punched it as hard as we could. This haphazard practice led to shredded skin where the straw pierced right through to the bone. When we got home we would have to remove the splinters with tweezers and sterilize the wounds with iodine…it was excruciating.

A generation later, by the time Kawasoe *sensei* was a student at the same university (Takushoku), things had changed little with regard to *makiwara* training for the students at the *karate* club. In Clive Layton's *Masao Kawasoe, 8ᵗʰ Dan: Reflections of a Shotokan Karate Master, The Early Years (1945–1975)*, he tells a similar story. On page 60, he says,

There were about six or seven makiwara lined up outside the dojo. We were required to face the makiwara every day—the seniors insisted. You must understand that what the seniors said was taken as law. I was used to training like this, but some of the other students were not. With the continual striking, the straw pads were covered with blood. The cuts on the fists—mine included I might add, such were the number of repetitions required—were not allowed to heal and they became wider and deeper. If you let up hitting the makiwara with full force, because of the pain, a senior, who would walk up and down behind you, would whack you with a bokken (wooden sword) to encourage you. Sometimes bits of straw would get embedded in the deep fissures and I can feel the excruciating pain now, as I talk about it, pulling them out. It was torturous, crazy training.

The writer continues,

This type of practice seems to have been implicit at Takushoku and had a history. Master Shiro Asano, who left Takushoku University some two years before Master Kawasoe began, recalled: "At Takushoku we could not stop. We had to carry on whatever the injury. There was not much concern for health and there was a lot of infection through cuts."

18. In a conversation with Shoshin Nagamine, founder of the *Matsubayashi* school of *Shorin ryu karate*, at his Kodokan *dojo* in Naha, Okinawa in 1992, he told me that in olden times (1800s to early 1900s?) men all over Okinawa would gather in backyards just to hit the *makiwara*. According to Nagamine *sensei*, who was eighty-five years old at the time of our conversation, these semi-social gatherings were attended by *karateka* and non-*karateka* alike.

    On a separate occasion, in the *dojo* of Ko Uehara, a highly respected teacher of *Goju ryu karate*, I was introduced to the two *makiwara* standing along the back wall close to the *dojo* entrance. One of them differed slightly from all others I had seen up to then in that attached to the wall at the rear of the *makiwara* was a small, plumb-line-like device. The weight could be moved closer to or further away from the back of the *makiwara*, and the idea was to hit the target hard enough for the head of the *makiwara* to penetrate through the air and set the small brass ball swinging. I was invited to try and try I did, several times. However, even with the weight only an inch or so from the back of the pad, I had no luck in moving the ball. Uehara *sensei* on the other hand had no trouble at all, even when he moved the weight right back to the wall.

19. In China, many books have been written over the centuries regarding the arts of war and personal combat. Sun Tzu's *Art of War* written in the sixth century is perhaps one of the better-known tomes dealing with conflict on a grand scale. The *Bubishi* (in Chinese, *Wu Bei Ji* and in English, *Account of Military Arts and Science*) is perhaps the best known for those seeking information relating to combat on a more personal level. The earliest copy dates from 1621, although there are a number of similar books with the same name. On Okinawa the *Bubishi* was considered the 'bible' of karate.

20. The IRKRS (International Ryukyu Karate Research Society), is a world-wide organization founded by Patrick McCarthy, a Canadian martial artist, now living in Australia. He is highly acclaimed for his in-depth research of *karate's* history and the teaching of older methods of training. A great deal of what is known in the West today, about the kind of training done by Okinawan *karateka* prior to the Second World War, is the result of his painstaking investigations into the past and willingness to share his discoveries with the wider *karate* community.

21. Placed in order of my first meetings with them are Seiko Kina (1984), Anichi Miyagi (1989), Shuichi Aragaki (1992), Eiichi Miyazato (1992), Seikichi Kinjo (1992), and Koshin Iha (1992).

Seiko Kina was a real gentleman and when I met him for the first time in his tiny *dojo* (the Junkokan) above his son's coffee shop at the back of the Heiwa-dori market in Naha the Okinawan capital, he made me feel very welcome. On that and subsequent meetings with him, he was always ready to show me the differences between *Naha-te* training ideas and those from *Shuri-te*. Friendly, helpful, and always willing to talk about the old days, I count myself very fortunate to have learned what little I did from him. By the time of my second visit to Okinawa, sadly, he had passed away.

Anichi Miyagi (no relation to Chojun) I met for the first and only time in San Diego, California, during the first Chojun Miyagi Memorial Festival, organized and presented by Morio Higaonna and his IOGKF (International Okinawan Goju ryu Karate Federation) organization in October 1989. I trained under him in a number of classes, but then so did many dozens of others at the same time, so I learned very little from him. Two years previously in 1987, when I took the test for 1st *Dan* in *Goju ryu* under Morio Higaonna in Tokyo, Anichi Miyagi also signed and stamped my certificate. He did write to me once, some years later, concerning a matter regarding Eiichi Miyazato, but my courteous reply made it clear I did not want to become involved in what I considered a matter between them.

I didn't get to train with **Shuichi Aragaki** when I met him at the Higaonna *dojo*; in fact he seemed slightly irritated that I was a student of Eiichi Miyazato, and so our meeting was not the one I had hoped for. As he had trained with Chojun Miyagi for only twenty-eight months before leaving Okinawa to live in Tokyo, a month before his teacher's death, I found his insights into Chojun Miyagi limited, and maybe it was this that gave cause to his irritation?

A student of his, my close friend Richard Barrett, introduced me to **Eiichi Miyazato** and from that first meeting I knew I had met someone special. I became his student and remained so until his death in December 1999. Just a few weeks before his passing he sent me a certificate awarding me a 6th *Dan*. It came out of the blue and was typical of his enigmatic character. He was often a man of few words, preferring instead to let his actions speak for him. He was much admired and is very sadly missed.

Seikichi Kinjo was training at the Jundokan *dojo* when I became a member there in 1992. Quiet and unassuming, and always ready to help, he is a wonderful example of the benefits of lifelong training. Even with a permanent tremor in his left arm, his strength during *kakie* (pushing hand training) often left me with burning muscles and a feeling that my arms would drop off at any moment. Sometimes he would stop me in mid-*kata* and show me an alternative way of doing a technique, or show me an application; his explanations often ended with "This Chojun *sensei*'s way!" He left the Jundokan *dojo* in 2006 but continues to train himself on a daily basis.

Although **Koshin Iha** was considered the most senior person in the Jundokan after Miyazato *sensei*, his presence, at least during my many visits there, was often sporadic. Most noticeable for teaching and sometimes training in his normal clothes, in the years following Miyazato *sensei*'s death he returned to wearing a *dogi* in the *dojo*. When I was introduced to him for the first time by Miyazato *sensei*, he seemed to take a dislike to me for some reason. I later discovered this was due, in part, to my having once been a student of Morio Higaonna. Nevertheless, in February 2004 I undertook a physical test for 7th *Dan* under his watchful gaze. Seven months later, a certificate arrived.

22. At that time my *dojo* stood in the backyard of my home in Perth, Western Australia. These days I live in Tasmania, and as before, my *dojo* stands adjacent to my home. This is the Okinawan way and, I believe, an important aspect of *karate* that is missing in today's business-like approach to running *karate* clubs and academies. It is not within the scope of this book to expand on this point further; suffice to say, I believe that when we are prepared to accept people into our *dojo* that we would not happily accept into our home, we change the very nature of the teacher and student relationship.

Glossary

The translation from Japanese to English is not precise; instead I have tried to convey the information necessary to understand the meaning behind the Japanese words. I have also refrained from listing the many hundreds of individual techniques found in karate. The prompts throughout the text and this list of general terms and commonly used words will, I'm sure, afford more than enough information to those unfamiliar with the terminology found in the dojo.

Terms Frequently Used in Traditional Karate

rei	Bow
waza	Technique
jodan	Upper area
chudan	Middle area
gedan	Lower area
zuki	Punch
uke	Block
uchi	Strike
keage	Snapping feeling
kekomi	Thrusting feeling
kimi	Focused feeling
muchimi (hogen)	Heavy, magnetic feeling
yoko	Side
hidari	Left
migi	Right
mae	Front/Forward
ushiro	Back/Behind
han	Half
han-mae	Half forward, usually referring to the position of the hips
yoi	Get ready/On guard
kamae	Any combat ready posture
hajime	Begin
yame	Stop

General Stances (Dachi)

Terms are listed in the order of progression from one stance to the next, starting with the feet together (*heisoku dachi*), moving outward and sideways to the feet being wide apart (*shiko dachi*), before stepping forward (*sanchin dachi* being the shortest step forward, *zenkutsu dachi* the longest). The other stances are used for specific reasons of either attack or defense, and finally the *embusen* is the floor plan of steps taken during a *kata*

dachi	Stance
heisoku dachi	Feet together
musubi dachi	Heels together, toes apart, V shape

heiko dachi	Natural posture with the feet about shoulder width apart
hachiji dachi	Same as *heiko dachi*, but with the feet turned slightly out
shiko dachi	Low stance/feet open, sometimes called horse riding stance
kiba dachi	Same as *shiko dachi*, but with the feet parallel
sanchin dachi	Hourglass stance, hips lowered/legs bent/front foot turned in
zenkutsu dachi	Forward stance, the length is twice that of a normal step
han-zenkutsu dachi	Half the length of *zenkutsu dachi*, one normal step in length
fudo dachi	Similar to *shiko dachi* but with a different weight distribution
kokutsu dachi	Back stance, weight distributed mostly on the rear leg
nekoashi dachi	Cat stance, rear leg bent/like a compressed spring
renoji dachi	Feet in a 10 o'clock position, front foot slightly forward
embusen	The pattern of steps or floor plan of directions taken in a *kata*

Types of Movements Used Frequently in Karate

tai sabaki	General term for 'body shifting'
tenshin	Another expression for indicating body movement
ayumi ashi	Normal stepping
yori ashi	Dragging the feet, a feeling like walking in ankle deep mud
suri ashi	Sliding step, pushing one leg quickly, then pulling the other
chakuchi	Replacing one foot with the other, like in a bench step up exercise

Common Hand, Arm, and Leg Parts Used in Karate

(Sorted from top part of the body to the tips of the toes.)

ude	Arm
te	Hand
seiken	Front of a fist, referring to the first two knuckles
ura	Back of the hand
tettsui	Opposite from the thumb side of hand when the fist is clenched; hammer fist
shuto	Side edge of the hand running from the wrist to little finger
haito	Opposite edge of the hand from *shuto*
nukite	Fingertips
ashi	Leg, but also means foot
hiza	Knee
koshi	Ball of foot
sokuto	Edge of foot running from the heel to the small toe
kakato	Heel
sokko	Instep
teisoku	Sole of the foot
tsumasaki	Tips of the toes

Other Terms From the Text

age	Rising
awase	Two handed
barai	Sweeping
bokken	Wooden sword
Bubishi	A Chinese martial arts book first written in 1621. "Account of Military Art and Science" (Chinese: *Wu Bei Ji*)
budo	Lit: Martial way. Deeper meaning: the way of stopping violence
budoka	Someone who studies the concept of *budo* through the practice of a martial art
bunbu ryodo	The way of the martial scholar. A person who trains their body for war and their mind for peace
bushi	In Okinawa – a gentleman warrior / In Japan – a samurai
empi	Old Japanese word for the elbow
furi	Whip-like action
gasshuku	Lit: Lodging together. Term used these days for a residential training course
geri	Kick
geta	Sandals or clogs
gyaku zuki	Reverse (as in the punch came off the reverse hip)
hantai	Opposite side...change sides!
hara	One's center, lower abdomen, area below the navel
heiza geri	Knee kick
hekite	Returning hand. The opposite hand to the one punching
hiji	Modern name for the elbow
hikei	Grasping
irimi	Entering, as in moving forward into an attack
karatedo	The way of the empty hand
kata	Form, the way something is done
kenpo	Way of the fist
kesage	A term used in *Shotokan karate* for a thrusting heel kick as in *kesage geri*
kiai	Spirit harmony, the coming together of mind, body, and spirit in the same moment. Commonly used these days as the name for the shout issued when executing a technique with full force
kigu undo	Another term for *hojo undo*
kobudo	Lit: Old martial ways. Today used to denote training with traditional Okinawan weapons
kori	A vital (nerve) point on the foot, just above the toes
kumite	Fighting
ma ai	Distance, between two or more people
mawashi	Swinging

mawate	Turning to face the opposite direction
migi sanchin dachi	Right leg forward *sanchin dachi*
Mook Jung	Chinese name for a 'wooden man' training tool similar to the *ude kitae*
Muk Yang Jong	(as above) An alternative Chinese name for the same training tool
nukite	Fingertip thrust
otomo	'O' means great, and 'tomo' comes from the word *tomodachi*, meaning friend. On a deeper level, to act with *otomo* is to develop your sense of attentiveness.
san dan gi	Three-step technique (step here refers to a position, not a walking kind of step)
sanchin	*San* – three, *Chin* – battles. In a broader sense, it is a training kata to find the harmony between the breath, the body and the mind
shin gi tai	Lit: spirit – technique - body
shotei	'Palm heel' the padded area at the wrist end of the open hand
suigetsu	A point on the body at the base of the sternum bone in the chest. In the West, we would call it our *solar plexus*
tanden	One's center, a point just below the navel
tensho	Name of a *kata* - Rotating palms
tora	Tiger
toudi	Old name for *karate* used in Okinawa
uraken	Back fist

Bibliography

Alexander, George W. *Okinawa: Island of Karate.* Lake Worth, FL: Yamazato Publications, 1991.

Bishop, Mark. *Okinawan Karate: Teachers, Styles and Secret Techniques.* 2nd ed. Boston, MA: Tuttle Publishing, 1999.

Bittmann, Heiko. *The Teachings of Karatedō.* Kanazawa, Japan: Heiko Bittmann Publishing, 2005.

Draeger, Donn F. and Robert W. Smith. *Comprehensive Asian Fighting Arts.* 4th ed. Tokyo and New York: Kodansha International, 1983.

Funakoshi, Gichin. *Tanpenshu; untold stories.* Compiled and translated by Patrick and Yuriko McCarthy. Brisbane, Australia: International Ryukyu Karate Research Society, 2004.

Harrison, Ernest John, *The Manual of Karate.* Translated from the Japanese, New York: Sterling Publication, 1966.

Higaonna, Morio. *Traditional Karatedo,* Vol. 1 in *Fundamental Techniques.* Tokyo: Minato Research/Japan Publications, 1985.

Higaonna, Morio. *The History of Karate – Okinawan Goju-ryu.* Westlake Village, CA: Dragon Books, 1996.

Hokama, Tetsuhiro. *Timeline of Karate History.* Translated by Joe Swift. Self-Published by Tetsuhiro Hokama. Nishihara, Okinawa: Ozato Print Co, 2007.

Hokama, Tetsuhiro and Matsu Kinjo. *Okinawa no Kobudo-gu, Tanren-dogu.* (in Japanese). Naha, Okinawa: Ryukyu Shinpo Newspaper Co., 1989.

Kanazawa, Hirokazu. *Shotokan Karate International Kata.* Vol. 2. Tokyo, Japan: S.K.I., 1982.

Kanazawa, Hirokazu. *Karate My Life.* Translated by Alex Bennett. Japan: Kendo World Publications Ltd, 2003.

Layton, Clive. *Conversations with Karate Masters.* Birkenhead, England: Ronin Publishing, 1988.

Layton, Clive. *Masao Kawasoe, 8th Dan: Recollections of a Shotokan Karate Master—The Early Years (1945-1975).* Llangefni, Wales: Mona Books (www.monabooks.co.uk), 2008.

Layton, Clive. *Shotokan Dawn.* Vol. 1. Llangefni, Wales: Mona Books (www.monabooks. co.uk), 2007.

Mattson, George E. *Uechiryu Karate-dō: Classical Chinese Okinawan Self-Defense.* Newton, MA: Peabody Publishing, 1974.

Mattson, George E. *The Way of Karate.* Rutland, VT and Tokyo: Charles E. Tuttle Co, 1963.

McKenna, Mario. *Okinawa Karate and Kobudo Blog,* (okinawakarateblog@blogspot.com) 2008.

McKenna, Mario. "The Myths and Facts Surrounding Higashionna Kanryo." *Dragon Times Magazine* 19 (2000).

Motobu, Choki. *Karate My Art.* 2nd ed. Compiled and translated from Japanese by Patrick and Yuriko McCarthy. Brisbane, Australia: International Ryukyu Karate Research Group, 2006.

Nagamine, Shoshin. *Tales of Okinawan Great Masters.* Translated by Patrick McCarthy, Rutland, VT: Tuttle Publishing, 1997.

Nakayama, Masatoshi. *Dynamic Karate: Instruction by the Master.* Translated by Herman Kauz. Tokyo, Palo Alto, CA: Kodansha International, 1966.

Okinawa Prefecture Board of Education. Okinawa *Karate "Kobudo"* Graph. Naha, Okinawa, 1995.

Plée, Henri D. *Vaincre ou mourir l'esprit et la technique du: Karate-Do.* Paris: Judo International, 1955.

Plée, Henri D. *Karate by Pictures.* London: W. Foulsham, 1962.

Plée, Henri D. *Karate: Beginner to Black Belt.* London: W. Foulsham, 1967.

Porta, John. "Supplementary Training for Miyagi Chojun's Goju Ryu Karate." *Journal of Asian Martial Arts* 5, no. 2 (1996).

Radi, Charles. "Speaking with Kinjo Hiroshi," *International Ryukyu Karate Research Society Journal*, Brisbane, Australia. 1st quarter ed. (2008): 38.

Ship, Ron. "Japan's First Karate and Kobudo Museum." *Fighting Arts International* 8, no. 5 (1988): 37.

Suzuki, Tatsuo. *Karate-Do.* London: Pelham Books, 1967.

Yagi, Meitoku. *The Life Drama of the Man, Meitoku.* (in Japanese). Naha, Okinawa: Wakanatsu-Sha, 2000.

Yokata, Kousaku. "Shotokan Karate Myths: The Makiwara." *Shotokan Karate Magazine* 97 (October 2008): 24.

Recommended websites and blogs

Yamada-san.blogspot.com (The blog of Sanzinsoo)
Okinawakarateblog.blogspot.com (The blog of Mario McKenna)
Karatejutsu.blogspot.com (The blog of Charles C. Gooding)
Chibanaproject.blogspot.com (The blog of Terry Garrett)
Koryu-uchinadi.com (Website for Patrick McCarthy)

Index

A

Achilles tendon 12
Adho Muka Svanasana 161
anchors 31
ankle weights 103
Aragaki, Shuichi 187
Arakaki, Seisho 176, 183
Art of War 186
Asano, Shiro 112, 186
ashi barai 137
auxiliary exercises 155
awase zuki 12
Azato, Yasutsune (Anko) 50, 130

B

back lift and stretch 166
balance 12, 13, 14, 84, 85, 99, 144, 165
bamboo bundle. *See* tou
barbells 184. *See Also tan*
bare hands 130
Barrett, Richard 187
baseball bat 181
Bhujangasana 161
blocking 152
blocking post. *See kakite bikei*
blocking practice 151
Bodhidharma 183
body, breath, and mind 37
body catch and push 162
body conditioning 3, 147
bokken 181, 185, 186
breath 19, 24, 27, 32, 40, 42, 43, 45, 46, 52,
   60, 62, 63, 66, 68, 71, 73, 80, 81, 83, 90,
   95, 113, 114, 143, 151, 156, 157, 160,
   164, 173
breath, body, and mind 66
breathing
   importance of 175
   nigiri gami 62
breathing patterns 19
Bubishi 176, 186
budo 179
budoka 179
bunbu ryodo 4
bunkai 7

bushi 4

C

calloused knuckles 113
calm 9
cat stretch 157, 161
ceramics 58
chiishi 184
   double handle 49
   lifting methods 38
   lifting single handle 38
   origins 35
   origins in Okinawa 35
children 176
chinte Shotokan 20, 143
Chuan-fa 2, 184
chudan haito uke 19
chudan hikei uke 150
chudan uchi uke 136
chudan uke 23, 24, 43, 82, 149, 151, 152
chudan zuki 118, 150, 152
climbing 173
conditioning 3, 7, 128, 147
construction notes
   double handle *chiishi* 58
   ishisashi 86
   jari bako 131
   kongoken 97
   makiagi 33
   makiwara 118
   nigiri gami 64
   single handle *chiishi* 47
   tan 75
   tetsu geta 102
   tou 125
   ude kitae 138

D

Daruma 183
dojos
   author's 187
   Okinawa 184
double handle *chiishi* 49
   exercises 51
Draeger, Donn 181
drills without tools 155

drop and thrust 159
dumbbell. *See ishisashi*
E
embusen 61, 71, 82
empi uchi 159
energy transfer 18, 160
explosive power 90, 92, 93, 101, 115
F
fingers 22, 177
fireman's lift and squat 165
Fuken fighting style 175
Funakoshi, Gichin 4, 5, 128, 130
   jari bako 127
furi uke 143
Fuzhou, China 182
G
gada 183
gar nal 183
gasshuku 155
gedan 135
gedan barai 136, 149, 152
gedan uke 151
gedan zuki 152
gekisai dai ni Goju ryu kata 63
gekisai kata 11, 12
geta 99, 102
Goju ryu, junbi undo exercises 9
Goju ryu karate 9, 87, 130, 175, 186
   muchimi 23
Goju ryu kata 17, 18, 19, 20, 24, 63, 176,
   184
Goju ryu kata kururunfa 14
Goju ryu kata seisan 12
Goodin, Charles C. 184
grabbing action 129
graveyards 184
grinding stones 35
gripping
   ishibukoro 168
   nigiri gami 59
   tou 124
gripping jars. *See nigiri gami*
grips 23
gyaku zuki 181
gyaku zuki punch 116

H
Hanashiro, Chomo 127
handgrip 168
hantai 143
hara 63, 157
Harada, Gojuro 181
harmony 71, 114
   body, breath, and mind 37
   chiishi 38
Harrison, E.J. 4
Hawaiian wrestlers 87
heavy bag 169
heiko dachi 11, 18, 19, 22, 24, 25, 27, 80, 92,
   93, 94, 151, 166
heiza geri 13, 100
hekite 117, 123
hidari jodan gyaku zuki 11
Higaonna, Kanryo 7, 175, 182, 184
Higaonna, Morio 51, 182, 183, 187
Higashionna. *See* Higaonna
hiji uchi 26
hiji uke 26
hikei uke 46, 144
Hironishi, Mononobu 5
Hiroshi, Kinjo 127
Ho, Chou Tsu 184
hojo undo 6
   decline in use of tools 3
   origins 175
   training 177
   training without tools 155
hojo undo training 128, 155, 179, 185
Hokama, Tetsuhiro 31, 183
I
Iha, Koshin 187
impact tools 105
impact training 147, 172
Indian tool training 183
Indian wrestlers 183
International Okinawan Goju ryu Karate
   Federation (IOGKF) 187
International Ryukyu Karate Research Society
   (IRKRS) 186
ippon uke barai 151
irimi 143

iron *geta* 103, 181
iron ring 168. *See* kongoken; *See* *tetsuwa*
iron sandal. *See* *tetsu geta*
iron tools 79
iron wheels 66
ishibukuro 168
ishisashi 79, 101, 184
    construction notes 86
    exercises 80
Itosu, Anko 130

J

jari bako 127
    construction notes 131
    exercises 129
jars 58. *See Also nigiri gami*
Jigen ryu 185
jodan 151
jodan age uke 151
jodan hidari tettsui uchi 143
jodan shuto uchi 11
jodan uke 152
jodan zuki 152
jori 183
junbi undo 6, 9
junbi undo exercise types 9

K

kakato geri 12
kakie 187
kakite bikei 141
    construction notes 145
    exercises 142
Kamata, Hiroshi 181
Kanazawa, Hirokazu 112, 141, 183, 185
karate 112
    earliest books 4
    early *hojo undo* training 4
    England 6
    Europe 5
    history 1
    hojo undo in Okinawa 6
    Japan 3
    Japanese vs. Okinawan 6
    makiwara 112
    Okinawan 7, 29, 179
    Okinawan *karatedo* 124

Shukokai 5
    sports 3
karate push-up 156
karate training 3, 4, 7, 65, 66, 128, 184
    auxiliary exercises 155
    mind activities 9
    other tools 167
    other training methods 173
kata 6, 176
kata training in Japan and Okinawa 6
Kawasoe, Masao 6, 112, 181, 186
kenpo 176
kesage geri 12
kiai 114, 115
kick bag 6, 124
kigu undo 1
kihon 6
kime 181
Kina, Seiko 187
Kinjo, Chinyei 184
Kinjo, Seikichi 187
knuckles 91, 112, 113, 156
kobudo 179
kobudo training 4
kongoken 88, 184
    construction notes 97
    exercises 89
kori 12
Ko, Ryu Ryu 183, 184
Ko-shan-kin 2
koshi 12, 93, 124, 162
koshi dachi 14
Kuang, Hsu Pao 1
Kumiai Jutsu 2
kumite 6, 176
Kurayoshi, Dr. 182
kururunfa Goju ryu kata 14, 63, 85
kushanku kata 2

L

Layton, Clive 181, 186
Lee, Bruce 182
leg lift and push 163
leg resistance 161
lifting
    chiishi 38

double handle *chiishi* 50
nigiri gami 59
single handle *chiishi* 38
lifting tools 29
lock (stone). *See ishisashi*
looms 31, 35
M
ma ai 141
Mabuni, Kenwa 4, 5
mae geri 12, 144, 181
makiage kigu. See makiagi
makiagi 30
construction notes 33
makiwara 112, 128, 177, 181, 184, 185, 186
construction notes 118
exercises 113
makiwara tsuki 185
mallakhamb 183
Matsubayashi school 186
Mattson, George E. 6, 181
mawashi uke 19, 20, 70
mawate 83
McCarthy, Patrick 184, 186
McKenna, Mario 182
mental training 9
migi sanchin dachi 154
mind, body, and breath 62
mind, body, and spirit 1, 73, 173, 179
mind, technique 114
Mirakian, Anthony 182
Miyagi, Anichi 187
Miyagi, Chojun 1, 5, 9, 79, 87, 130, 155,
175, 184, 187
Miyazato, Eiichi 79, 187
Mook Jung 135
muchimi 23, 62, 154
Muk Yang Jong 135
muscles
chiishi use 37
junbi undo 9
latissimus dorsi 81
musubi dachi 14
N
Nagamine, Shoshin 186
Nagoya, Sagenta 2
Naha-te 128, 187

Naha-te kata 67
naihanchin Shuri-te kata 67
nail *jori* 183
Nakasone, Genwa 4
Nakayama, Masatoshi 5, 6
Nakayama, Masyoshi 181
nekoashi dachi 134
nigiri gami 58, 184
construction notes 64
exercises 61
gripping 59
lifting 59
nukite 122, 123, 129, 181
O
Obata, Isao 181
Okinawa
ceramics 58
fighting arts 1
large jars 58
stones 79
tales 130
Okinawan karate 29, 179
one-step blocking practice. *See ippon uke
barai*
Oshiro, Chojo 127
162
Oya, Reikichi 4
P
Pangai Noon ryu 124
Plée, Henri D. 5, 181
pounding post 134
preparation exercises 9
punches 113, 114
makiwara 118
punching bags 185
push and body catch 162
push and leg lift 163
pushing hand training 187
push-ups 91, 156
R
Radi, Charles 127
reeds 123
rice 23
rocks 49
roller 170
running 173

S

saifa Goju ryu kata 18, 20, 63, 143
saifa kata 11
sanchin bar 171
sanchin dachi 11, 31, 60, 62, 63, 71, 72, 74, 82, 152
sanchin dai ni Goju ryu kata 18
sanchin double chudan uke 32
sanchin kata 19, 24, 59, 60, 61, 63, 71, 81, 82, 176
san dan gi 152
sandan uke barai 152
sand box. *See jari bako*
sanseiru Goju ryu kata 85
sanseiru kata 18
sanseiru Naha-te kata 67
sashi 80, 81, 82, 83, 84, 85
sashi ishi 50
seiken 181
seipai Goju ryu kata 18, 26, 63
seisan Goju ryu kata 18, 63, 85
seisan kata 12
seiyunchin
   Goju ryu kata 17, 18
   Naha-te kata 67
Senzuikyo 183
Shaolin boxing 183
Shaolin-szu 183
shiko dachi 15, 16, 18, 26, 37, 39, 40, 42, 43, 44, 45, 51, 52, 53, 67, 68, 69, 73, 81, 89, 90, 129, 151, 152, 159, 163, 165
shime 181
shin gi tai 179
Shito ryu 4
shock 147. *See Also* impact tools
Shohei ryu 124
Shorin ryu karate 2, 184, 186
shotei uchi 137, 159
shotei uke 142
Shotokan karate 4, 5, 127
   myths 184
Shotokan kata unsu 12
Shukokai Karate Union 5
Shuri-te 128, 187
Shuri-te kata 67
Shushiwa 184

shuto uchi 117
single handle *chiishi*
   construction notes 47
   exercises 40
skipping 173
Sokon, Matsumura 184
spear-hand strikes 122
spins 16
sports karate 3
spring bar 171
squat and fireman's lift 165
squats 14, 163
stamina 9
stand-ups 164
stone lock. *See ishisashi*
stones 31, 35, 66, 79
stone sack 168
straw rope 112
straw splinters 112
strength 7, 9, 37, 41
   auxilliary exercises 155
   chiishi 46
   ishibukuro 168
   jari bako grip 130
   kongoken 88
   legs 17
   tan 65
   tetsu geta 99
   toes 11, 14
strength stones. *See chiishi*
stretch and back lift 166
stretches 16, 157
   junbi undo 9
striking post. *See makiwara*
sugar cane 123
suigetsu point 118
sumtola 183
Sun Tzu 186
suparinpei Goju ryu kata 12, 18, 63
suri ashi 63
Suzuki, Tatsuo 6
swimming 173
swings 21

T

tai sabaki 63, 95, 143
taketaba. See tou

tan 184
    construction notes 75
    exercises 67
Tana, Mr. 182
tanden 24, 63, 83, 90, 93
Tani, Chojiro 5
Tani Ha Shito ryu 5
tapping stick 172
Tasmania 187
teisoku 11, 62
tekki Shuri-te kata 67
tendons 9
tensho kata 176
tetsu geta 99
    construction notes 102
    exercises 100
tetsuwa 168
tettsui uchi 134
thrust and drop 159
Tobe, Yoshihiro 2
toes 11, 12, 14, 177
    control tactics 11
    tetsu geta 99
Tokashiki, Iken 182
Tomari-te 128
tools 179
    drills without 155
    Indian 183
    other 167
tora uchi 19, 69
torso wheel 170
tou 122, 184
    construction notes 125
    exercises 123
    origins 123
traditional training 6, 66, 185
training partner
    auxiliary exercises 156
    body catch and push 162
    fireman's squat and lift 165
    heavy squats 163
    hojo undo 147
    kongoken 92, 96
    leg lift and push 163
    leg resistance 161

resistance punching 160
    stand-ups 164
    ude tanren 148
trinity of *shin gi tai* (mind, body, spirit) 1, 73, 173, 179
Tsukunesu Jutsu 2
Tsuyama sensei 181
twisting 11
two-person conditioning exercises 147

UVW
ude kitae 134
    construction notes 138
    exercises 136
    Okinawan and Chinese 135
ude tanren 147
    exercises 149
Uechi, Kanbun 184
Uechi, Kanei 181
Uechi ryu 124, 181
Uechi ryu kata 184
Uehara, Ko 186
unsu Shotokan kata 12
uraken 116, 142
Vickers, David 5
Wado ryu karate 6
warm-up exercises 9, 10
weaving 183
weight transfer 16, 17
wheel 170
wooden-man 135
wrestlers 35, 87
wrist rotation 154
XYZ
Xian, Xie Zhong 183, 184
Xi Shui Jin 183
Yabu, Master 176
Yamani ryu bojutsu 184
Yi Jing Jin 183
yoga 157
yoi 60
Yokata, Kousaku 184
yoko geri 11, 85
zenkutsu dachi 83, 101, 116

About the Author

Michael Clarke grew up in Manchester, in the heart of England's industrial North. Leaving school at 15 years of age, fairly well educated but without qualifications, frustration with his position in life soon began to manifest in anti-social and violent behavior. His downward spiral culminated in jail time, and it was from here that he began his climb back to propriety. Thirty-five years later, he is a different person. A prolific essayist, recognized around the world for his writings on the philosophical aspects of *karate* that underpin the physical training, his commentaries have appeared in magazines since 1985 in America, Australia, England, Japan, New Zealand, and Portugal. Upon request, his articles have been posted on Web sites where some have been translated into Spanish, Portuguese, Dutch, French, and Japanese.

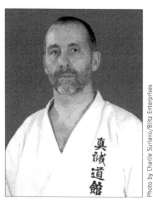

Also known for his interviewing skills, Michael has throughout the past twenty-five years published over forty interviews, many with teachers of international renown, such as the present *Doshu* of *Aikido*, Moriteru Ueshiba; Hirokazu Kanazawa of *Shotokan;* Morio Higaonna of *Goju Ryu*; and Tatsuo Suzuki of *Wado ryu*, to name but a few. As well, he has interviewed other famous instructors, and many who are not. Nine of his early interviews were published in his second book, *Budo Master: Paths to a Far Mountain;* and his autobiographical accounts of life, travel, and training in his book *Roaring Silence* and its companion volume *Small Steps Forward* have given inspiration to many.

These days Michael lives quietly with his wife, Kathy, high on a hill overlooking a bend in the river Tamar, in Northern Tasmania. Surrounded by natural bush land, he practices *karate* and *kobudo* in the small *dojo* attached to his home and spends the rest of his time reading, writing, walking in the forest surrounding his home, and watching science fiction movies. He can be contacted at www.shinseidokandojo.blogspot.com.

BOOKS FROM YMAA

ADVANCING IN TAE KWON DO	B072X
ANALYSIS OF SHAOLIN CHIN NA 2ND ED	B0002
ANCIENT CHINESE WEAPONS	B671
ART OF HOJO UNDO	B1361
BAGUAZHANG 2ND ED.	B1132
CARDIO KICKBOXING ELITE	B922
CHIN NA IN GROUND FIGHTING	B663
CHINESE FAST WRESTLING	B493
CHINESE TUI NA MASSAGE	B043
CHOJUN	B2535
COMPREHENSIVE APPLICATIONS OF SHAOLIN CHIN NA	B36X
CUTTING SEASON—A XENON PEARL MARTIAL ARTS THRILLER	B1309
DESHI—A CONNOR BURKE MARTIAL ARTS THRILLER	E2481
DIRTY GROUND	B2115
DUKKHA, THE SUFFERING—AN EYE FOR AN EYE	B2269
EIGHT SIMPLE QIGONG EXERCISES FOR HEALTH, 2ND ED.	B523
ESSENCE OF SHAOLIN WHITE CRANE	B353
ESSENCE OF TAIJI QIGONG, 2ND ED.	B639
FACING VIOLENCE	B2139
FIGHTING ARTS	B213
FORCE DECISIONS—A CITIZENS GUIDE	B2436
INSIDE TAI CHI	B108
KAGE—THE SHADOW A CONNOR BURKE MARTIAL ARTS THRILLER	B2108
KATA AND THE TRANSMISSION OF KNOWLEDGE	B0266
KRAV MAGA—WEAPON DEFENSES	B2405
LITTLE BLACK BOOK OF VIOLENCE	B1293
MARTIAL ARTS ATHLETE	B655
MARTIAL ARTS INSTRUCTION	B024X
MARTIAL WAY AND ITS VIRTUES	B698
MASK OF THE KING	B114
MEDITATIONS ON VIOLENCE	B1187
MUGAI RYU	B183
NATURAL HEALING WITH QIGONG	B0010
NORTHERN SHAOLIN SWORD, 2ND ED.	B85X
OKINAWA'S COMPLETE KARATE SYSTEM—ISSHIN RYU	B914
POWER BODY	B760
PRINCIPLES OF TRADITIONAL CHINESE MEDICINE	B99X
QIGONG FOR HEALTH & MARTIAL ARTS 2ND ED.	B574
QIGONG FOR LIVING	B116
QIGONG FOR TREATING COMMON AILMENTS	B701
QIGONG MASSAGE	B0487
QIGONG MEDITATION—EMBRYONIC BREATHING	B736
QIGONG MEDITATION—SMALL CIRCULATION	B0673
QIGONG, THE SECRET OF YOUTH—DA MO'S CLASSICS	B841
QUIET TEACHER—A XENON PEARL MARTIAL ARTS THRILLER	B1262
RAVEN'S WARRIOR	B2580
ROOT OF CHINESE QIGONG, 2ND ED.	B507
SCALING FORCE	B2504
SENSEI—A CONNOR BURKE MARTIAL ARTS THRILLER	E2474
SHIHAN TE—THE BUNKAI OF KATA	B884
SHIN GI TAI—KARATE TRAINING FOR BODY, MIND, AND SPIRIT	B2177
SIMPLE CHINESE MEDICINE	B1248
SUNRISE TAI CHI	B0838
SURVIVING ARMED ASSAULTS	B0711
TAE KWON DO—THE KOREAN MARTIAL ART	B0869
TAEKWONDO BLACK BELT POOMSAE	B1286
TAEKWONDO—ANCIENT WISDOM FOR THE MODERN WARRIOR	B930
TAEKWONDO—DEFENSES AGAINST WEAPONS	B2276
TAEKWONDO—SPIRIT AND PRACTICE	B221
TAI CHI BALL QIGONG—FOR HEALTH AND MARTIAL ARTS	B1996
TAI CHI BOOK	B647
TAI CHI CHUAN—24 & 48 POSTURES	B337
TAI CHI CHUAN CLASSICAL YANG STYLE (REVISED EDITION)	B2009
TAI CHI CHUAN MARTIAL APPLICATIONS, 2ND ED.	B442
TAI CHI CONNECTIONS	B0320
TAI CHI DYNAMICS	B1163
TAI CHI SECRETS OF THE ANCIENT MASTERS	B71X
TAI CHI SECRETS OF THE WU & LI STYLES	B981
TAI CHI SECRETS OF THE YANG STYLE	B094
TAI CHI THEORY & MARTIAL POWER, 2ND ED.	B434
TAI CHI WALKING	B23X
TAIJI CHIN NA	B378
TAIJI SWORD—CLASSICAL YANG STYLE	B744
TAIJIQUAN THEORY OF DR. YANG, JWING-MING	B432
TRADITIONAL CHINESE HEALTH SECRETS	B892

more products available from . . .

YMAA Publication Center, Inc. 楊氏東方文化出版中心

1-800-669-8892 • info@ymaa.com • www.ymaa.com

BOOKS FROM YMAA (continued)

TRADITIONAL TAEKWONDO	B0665
WAY OF KATA	B0584
WAY OF KENDO AND KENJITSU	B0029
WAY OF SANCHIN KATA	B0845
WAY TO BLACK BELT	B0852
WESTERN HERBS FOR MARTIAL ARTISTS	B1972
WILD GOOSE QIGONG	B787
WOMAN'S QIGONG GUIDE	B833
XINGYIQUAN, 2ND ED.	B416

DVDS FROM YMAA

ADVANCED PRACTICAL CHIN NA IN-DEPTH	D1224
ANALYSIS OF SHAOLIN CHIN NA	D0231
BAGUAZHANG—EMEI BAGUAZHANG	D0649
CHEN STYLE TAIJIQUAN	D0819
CHIN NA IN-DEPTH COURSES 1—4	D602
CHIN NA IN-DEPTH COURSES 5—8	D610
CHIN NA IN-DEPTH COURSES 9—12	D629
EIGHT SIMPLE QIGONG EXERCISES FOR HEALTH	D0037
ESSENCE OF TAIJI QIGONG	D0215
FACING VIOLENCE—7 THINGS A MARTIAL ARTIST MUST KNOW	D2283
FIVE ANIMAL SPORTS	D1106
KNIFE DEFENSE—TRADITIONAL TECHNIQUES AGAINST A DAGGER	D1156
KUNG FU BODY CONDITIONING 1	D2085
KUNG FU BODY CONDITIONING 2	D2290
KUNG FU FOR KIDS	D1880
LOGIC OF VIOLENCE	D2351
NORTHERN SHAOLIN SWORD —SAN CAI JIAN, KUN WU JIAN, QI MEN JIAN	D1194
QIGONG FOR HEALING	D2320
QIGONG FOR LONGEVITY	D2092
QIGONG FOR WOMEN	D2566
SABER FUNDAMENTAL TRAINING	D1088
SHAOLIN KUNG FU FUNDAMENTAL TRAINING—COURSES 1 & 2	D0436
SHAOLIN LONG FIST KUNG FU—BASIC SEQUENCES	D661
SHAOLIN LONG FIST KUNG FU—INTERMEDIATE SEQUENCES	D1071
SHAOLIN LONG FIST KUNG FU—ADVANCED SEQUENCES 1	D2061
SHAOLIN LONG FIST KUNG FU—ADVANCED SEQUENCES 2	D2313
SHAOLIN SABER—BASIC SEQUENCES	D0616
SHAOLIN STAFF—BASIC SEQUENCES	D0920
SHAOLIN WHITE CRANE GONG FU BASIC TRAINING—COURSES 1 & 2	D599
SHAOLIN WHITE CRANE GONG FU BASIC TRAINING—COURSES 3 & 4	D0784
SHUAI JIAO—KUNG FU WRESTLING	D1149
SIMPLE QIGONG EXERCISES FOR ARTHRITIS RELIEF	D0890
SIMPLE QIGONG EXERCISES FOR BACK PAIN RELIEF	D0883
SIMPLIFIED TAI CHI CHUAN—24 & 48 POSTURES	D0630
SUNRISE TAI CHI	D0274
SUNSET TAI CHI	D0760
SWORD—FUNDAMENTAL TRAINING	D1095
TAI CHI BALL QIGONG—COURSES 1 & 2	D0517
TAI CHI BALL QIGONG—COURSES 3 & 4	D0777
TAI CHI CHUAN CLASSICAL YANG STYLE	D645
TAI CHI CONNECTIONS	D0444
TAI CHI ENERGY PATTERNS	D0525
TAI CHI FIGHTING SET	D0509
TAI CHI PUSHING HANDS—COURSES 1 & 2	D0495
TAI CHI PUSHING HANDS—COURSES 3 & 4	D0681
TAI CHI SWORD—CLASSICAL YANG STYLE	D0452
TAIJI & SHAOLIN STAFF—FUNDAMENTAL TRAINING	D0906
TAIJI CHIN NA IN-DEPTH	D0463
TAIJI 37 POSTURES MARTIAL APPLICATIONS	D1057
TAIJI SABER CLASSICAL YANG STYLE	D1026
TAIJI WRESTLING	D1064
UNDERSTANDING QIGONG 1—WHAT IS QI? • HUMAN QI CIRCULATORY SYSTEM	D069X
UNDERSTANDING QIGONG 2—KEY POINTS • QIGONG BREATHING	D0418
UNDERSTANDING QIGONG 3—EMBRYONIC BREATHING	D0555
UNDERSTANDING QIGONG 4—FOUR SEASONS QIGONG	D0562
UNDERSTANDING QIGONG 5—SMALL CIRCULATION	D0753
UNDERSTANDING QIGONG 6—MARTIAL QIGONG BREATHING	D0913
WHITE CRANE HARD & SOFT QIGONG	D637
WUDANG KUNG FU—FUNDAMENTAL TRAINING	D1316
WUDANG SWORD	D1903
WUDANG TAIJIQUAN	D1217
XINGYIQUAN	D1200
YANG TAI CHI FOR BEGINNERS	D2306
YMAA 25 YEAR ANNIVERSARY DVD	D0708

more products available from . . .
YMAA Publication Center, Inc. 楊氏東方文化出版中心

1-800-669-8892 • info@ymaa.com • www.ymaa.com